Immediate Decisions

For Birth in any Trimester

Based on the pages of *still*birthday

A pregnancy loss is still a birthday

DEDICATION

To your baby or babies, with love for them and reverence for their legacy,
from my own bereaved mother's heart, and from yours.
We are in this together, and you are not alone.

Your baby's name

CONTENTS

ACKNOWLEDGMENTS

I acknowledge you.
This journey is real, and it is difficult.
Please visit stillbirthday for more comprehensive support prior to, during and after birth in any trimester.

This handbook is simply the most basic of possible birth preparation as you embark on the hardest journey of your life.

A Pregnancy Loss is Still a Birthday

Please know that you are not alone.
There are professionally trained birth &
bereavement doulas who are prepared to come
alongside you on this journey.

Just visit:

www.stillbirthday.com/find-doula

The following are the most frequently visited pages
at stillbirthday, a global resource that has been
translated into multiple languages to provide
support to more than one million families each year.

These pages are a compilation of items and basic
expectations to prepare yourself for what to
possibly expect in the earliest days of experiencing
pregnancy and infant loss.

These are based on the information current to 2014
but this information is updated regularly.

Please visit www.stillbirthday.com.

A Pregnancy Loss is Still a Birthday

THE EARLIEST WORDS

The words spoken to you in the earliest moments can ring as the most memorable, for better or for worse. Medical terminology is an important foundation for a continuity of language amongst obstetricians, ultrasound technicians, nurses and other medical staff. But if you're wanting to understand a little bit more, just what those words mean that medically describe such a personal experience, the following pages may serve to translate some of the language in a way that is informative and validating.

IN MY OWN WORDS
This is how I define my own experience

When I learned I was pregnant:

_____

_____

_____

Experiences in this pregnancy:

_____

_____

_____

When I learned my baby was not alive:

_____

_____

_____

What my heart is saying:

_____

_____

_____

My spiritual beliefs say:

_____

_____

_____

How my spouse is feeling or responding:

_____

_____

_____

My biggest fears or feelings right now:

_____

_____

_____

One person I can call or visit any time to be reminded that I am loved:

_____

_____

_____

One favorite thing I can enjoy to be reminded of pleasurable things:

_____

_____

_____

Three resources I can utilize at any time for support:

_____

_____

_____

For physical support, these are local nurses, midwives, hospitals I trust:

_____

_____

_____

IN CASE OF EMERGENCY, I CAN CALL

_____

_____

_____

- First Candle offers 24/7 phone support in English and Spanish: 800.221.7437 lori@firstcandle.org

- COPEline offers phone support (leave a message if it's after hours and a volunteer will call you back): 516.364.COPE (2673)

- National Council of Jewish Women free phone support (212) 687-5030 ext. 28 or at plsp@ncjwny.org

- US National Suicide Prevention Hotline offers 24/7 confidential support: 800.273.TALK

- Grassroots Crisis Hotline: 410.531.6677

- SIDS Hotline (Sudden Infant Death Syndrome): 800.232.SIDS (7437)

- Focus on the Family Christian counseling hotline and resources

- **Canada** Crisis Line: 888.322.3019

- **Canada** Suicide Prevention Hotline: 877.435.7170

MY FEELINGS

_____
_____
_____
_____
_____
_____
_____
_____
_____
_____
_____
_____
_____
_____
_____
_____
_____
_____
_____
_____
_____
_____
_____
_____
_____
_____
_____
_____
_____
_____

_____

_____

_____

_____

_____

_____

_____

_____

_____

_____

_____

_____

_____

_____

_____

_____

_____

_____

_____

_____

_____

_____

_____

_____

_____

_____

_____

_____

_____

_____

THIS IS MY STORY

ZEROES COUNT

Those things that may never be in this life, the wishes we have, the hopes that are lost, these things still count. Even unseen, they make up who we are. Use this circle to create a womandala. In a safe space, connect with your feelings and then use the colors that speak to you.

When you are done, consider sharing your art with someone you love, and treat yourself to something special for completing your healing activity.

MEDICAL TERMINOLOGY EXPLAINED

CHEMICAL PREGNANCY

If you have begun to miscarry, and hadn't yet been able to hear your baby's heartbeat with a doppler, your doctor might have said that you are having a chemical pregnancy. This means that it's a very early miscarriage.

Related: please read our Honoring Uncertainty

This very early miscarriage—or the name of it—doesn't make your baby any less real. At 5 weeks gestation, just about the time you may have found out that you were pregnant, your baby was about the size of a sesame seed. And, at 5 weeks gestation, your tiny baby's heart has already begun to beat. It's just too small to be heard on a Doppler.

While identifying your baby at this stage is probably just not going to happen, because of everything that is delivered during the miscarriage, including uterine lining and lots of blood, your baby is real. Your feelings about your baby are real.

You will likely have a natural miscarriage, or natural delivery. Rarely, artificial induction or a D&C may be recommended. You can learn about these different birth methods here:

- natural delivery

- artificial induction (medication)

- D&C

You are invited to share your story here as well: please remember that sharing your story at stillbirthday is a way to express your feelings and share your experiences with other mothers – it is not to diagnose, treat or answer any medical questions.

You might visit our farewell celebrations for ideas to celebrate your baby.

HONORING UNCERTAINTY

Something happened. Something was... different.

You came to stillbirthday, you looked through our list of losses that we support, read a few of their descriptions – in particular, Chemical Pregnancy.

You looked at some of the photos we hold here at stillbirthday.

But... you're just not sure.

Everything seemed to happen so fast:

You felt pregnant, and then all of a sudden, you were met with blood.

Maybe lots of blood, and maybe with deeply painful cramping.

No real pregnancy test, there just wasn't time.

This was... something different.

There are many reasons why your cycle might change, even abruptly.

Sudden stress, including financial, social, or marital stress might impact your menstrual cycle.

Deep and longstanding stress might also impact your menstrual cycle.

Nutrition and self care also might have an impact.

Some mothers report a change in menstrual cycle after a big move, and there is something to be said for large sorority-type events that have a strong emphasis on women or motherhood. Examples might include women's rape survivor rallies, sexual trafficking fundraising or women's rights in childbirth conferences.

These things and more might have an otherwise unexplained change in your menstrual cycle.

Additionally, through our season of our menstruation, it is entirely possible, and even medically normal, to have an occasional menstrual cycle that is simply different.

And by different, any number of experiences might occur:

Your menstrual cycle might appear later, sooner, lighter or heavier than you usually experience.

If you have discussed these things with your doctor or midwife and still just feel unsure about what you experienced,

please know that here at stillbirthday, we honor your uncertainty.

The feeling of uncertainty isn't easier and it surely isn't simpler than bereavement.

Many mothers will resolve themselves to
"Well, I'll never know this side of eternity."

And that can be a lonely, painful place to be. Please know, you aren't alone.

And in a time that seems so very fast moving, with answers for most things readily available, even for early pregnancy tests, it can seem frustrating and disappointing not to have a certain answer.

If you believe you may have experienced loss but don't have anything to "prove" it, we validate you.

You are invited to share your story here as well: please remember that sharing your story at stillbirthday is a way to express your feelings and share your experiences with other mothers – it is not to diagnose, treat or answer any medical questions.

You might visit our farewell celebrations for ideas to celebrate your "Maybe Baby".

BLIGHTED OVUM

A blighted ovum means that a fertilized egg has attached itself to your uterine wall, but the embryo (baby) did not develop. Cells developed to form the placenta and the amniotic sac, but not the embryo itself.

While a positive pregnancy test detects the placenta hormones (not an actual baby), finding out that you are pregnant can be the beginning of hopes, aspirations and joy.

With a blighted ovum, your body may display signs of pregnancy, and may actually sustain the life of the growing placenta for a short time. You may not know you have a blighted ovum until an ultrasound confirms it, or you may miscarry naturally before an ultrasound is performed.

The fact that a blighted ovum does not result in a baby can be equally–if not more–devastating than any other kind of miscarriage.

Finding out what to expect from your recommended birth method (listed below), and allowing yourself to experience healthy grief with a farewell celebration can be very useful and positive for you.

Please also utilize long term support services and emotional/spiritual health support services listed here in this website.

It is also very important to reach out, and tell others about your story. Please consider sharing your experience with us here and reading the stories shared here by other mothers who've experienced loss through blighted ovum.

We'd be so honored to learn from you and to cry with you.

Birth Methods:

- natural miscarriage

- D&C

We also hold photos of what you might expect to see or your blighted ovum to look like.

MOLAR PREGNANCY

There are two types of molar pregnancy:

Complete molar pregnancy. An egg with no genetic information is fertilized by a sperm. The sperm grows on its own, but it can only become a growth of placental tissue (hence a positive pregnancy test) and cannot become a fetus. In a complete mole, all of the fertilized egg's chromosomes (tiny thread-like structures in cells that carry genes) come from the father. Normally, half come from the father and half from the mother. In a complete mole, shortly after fertilization, the chromosomes from the mother's egg are lost or inactivated, and those from the father are duplicated. As this tissue grows, it looks a bit like a cluster of grapes. This cluster of tissue can very rapidly fill the uterus.

Partial molar pregnancy. An egg is fertilized by two sperm. If an abnormal embryo does begin to develop, it will quickly die because of the rapidly growing mass of abnormal tissue filling your uterus. In most cases of partial mole, the mother's 23 chromosomes remain, but there are two sets of chromosomes from the father (so the embryo has 69 chromosomes instead of the normal 46). This can happen when the chromosomes from the father are duplicated or if two sperm fertilize an egg.

Molar pregnancy poses a threat to the pregnant woman because it can occasionally result in a rare pregnancy-related form of cancer called choriocarcinoma (see end of document).

Molar pregnancy is assessed with a pelvic exam and ultrasound. The abnormal placenta mass will have a clustered, grape like appearance.

For these and other serious medical risks, the molar pregnancy is immediately ended with medical support. This is generally done with a D&C. Afterward, you will have regular blood tests to look for signs of trophoblastic disease. These blood tests will be done over the next 6 to 12 months. Your doctor will caution you that you will need to use birth control for the next 6 to 12 months so that you don't get pregnant. It is very important to see your doctor for all follow-up visits.

While a positive pregnancy test detects the placenta hormones (not an actual baby), finding out that you are pregnant can be the beginning of a hopes, aspirations and joy.

"THE FACT THAT A (COMPLETE) MOLAR PREGNANCY DOES NOT RESULT IN A BABY (OR, TWINS) CAN BE EQUALLY–IF NOT MORE–DEVASTATING THAN ANY OTHER KIND OF MISCARRIAGE.

PLEASE BE GENTLE ON YOURSELF AND KNOW THAT YOUR LOSS IS WORTHY TO GRIEVE."

- STILLBIRTHDAY MOTHER

Finding out what to expect from a D&C, and allowing yourself to experience healthy grief with a farewell celebration can be very useful and positive for you.

Please also utilize long term support services and emotional/spiritual health support services listed here in this website.

It is also very important to reach out, and tell others about your story. Please consider sharing your experience with us here, and reading the stories shared here by other mothers who've experienced molar pregnancy.

We'd be so honored to learn from you and to cry with you.

We hold photos of what a molar pregnancy may look like.

THREATENED MISCARRIAGE

If your doctor told you that you are having a threatened miscarriage, you should know:

Many mothers with threatened miscarriage go on to have a complete pregnancy.

It is better to find and treat health problems (particularly systemic ones) before you get pregnant than to wait until you're already pregnant.

Miscarriages are less likely if you receive early, comprehensive *prenatal care* and avoid environmental hazards such as x-rays, drugs and alcohol, high levels of caffeine, and infectious diseases. Being obese or having uncontrolled diabetes can increase your risk for miscarriage.

The use of *progesterone* is controversial. It might relax smooth muscles, including the muscles of the uterus. However, it also might increase the risk of an incomplete miscarriage or an abnormal pregnancy. Unless there is a luteal phase defect, progesterone should not be used.

The use of *false unicorn root* (or other herbs such as *cramp bark)* is also controversial. It is said to help "normalize" gynecological concerns with the uterus, including preventing miscarriage. This native US herb is said to help facilitate the release of hormones by the ovaries. Despite the claims to prevent miscarriage, there are warnings against using this herb in pregnancy. Please consult with your medical provider before attempting to use any herbs or other non-medical resources to sustain your pregnancy.

You may be told to *avoid or restrict some forms of activity*. Not having sexual intercourse is usually recommended until the warning signs have disappeared.

Remember A+B+C = abdominal pain, bleeding, cramping. These three *together* are signs of a probable miscarriage.

Are you experiencing additional signs of miscarriage?

We also have information in our Getting Pregnant Again section that may prove helpful to you in this pregnancy – things that are encouraging, and other non-medical things you might consider.

You are invited to share your story here as well: please remember that sharing your story at stillbirthday is a way to express your feelings and share your experiences with other mothers – it is not to diagnose, treat or answer any medical questions.

INEVITABLE OR INCOMPLETE MISCARRIAGE

An inevitable miscarriage is different from a threatened miscarriage, in that with an inevitable miscarriage, your baby will most certainly be born via miscarriage.

There are two situations that result in an inevitable (or incomplete) miscarriage:

- Your cervical opening begins to dilate (open) and you are having vaginal bleeding (see our article on signs of miscarriage). This means that your body is beginning to deliver your baby.
- Your baby has not developed (stayed the same size) over a two week period. Your baby's heartrate may be slowing, or have completely stopped.

An inevitable miscarriage might be first discovered by ultrasound at a routine doctor appointment, or if you are experiencing possible symptoms of miscarriage you may visit your OB or your emergency room for confirmation. The emergency room experience is often considered very unpleasant, but it may be needed. If you visit your local emergency room, consider these tips:

- let the staff know immediately that you believe you may be miscarrying
- ask about their bereavement support, including staff and materials
- ask if there is a women's, laboring, or miscarriage room within the emergency room, or if you can be transferred to the labor and delivery level if that is what you'd prefer. Once on the L&D level, ask for a room away from other mothers.

- you may need to fill your bladder to help locate your baby on ultrasound. Ask about drinking water, and curling on your side, rather than recieving a catheter. If one is needed, ask about what to expect once it is removed (you may see some blood in your urine, and you may be sore for several hours or longer).
- if you give birth to your baby in the emergency room, inquire of your personal options. Visit our early pregnancy hospital birth plan for more details. Understand navigating hospital policies, including genetic testing, returning your baby's physical form back to you after any testing, and any other questions you have.

If your baby is *younger* than about 12 weeks gestation, you may be given three options for delivery:
- natural delivery
- artificial induction (medication)
- D&C

If your baby is *older* than about 12 weeks gestation (about the beginning of the second trimester), you may be given these options for delivery:
- artificial induction (medication)
- D&C
- D&E

You are invited to share your story here as well: please remember that sharing your story at stillbirthday is a way to express your feelings and share your experiences with other mothers – it is not to diagnose, treat or answer any medical questions.

You might visit our farewell celebrations for ideas to celebrate your baby.

MISSED OR SILENT MISCARRIAGE

If your doctor told you that your baby's heart has stopped beating, you may be experiencing a missed miscarriage or an incomplete miscarriage.

You may have just found out that your baby's heart actually stopped beating several days ago (or a couple of weeks ago) and you are just now beginning to see the earliest signs of delivery (see symptoms of a miscarriage for a complete listing, but includes seeing blood and/or pieces of tissue passing from your vagina).

A missed miscarriage occurs when your baby has already died, but the actual birthing process either has not yet begun or isn't fully complete.

If your baby is *younger* than about 12 weeks gestation, you may be given three options for delivery:

- natural delivery
- artificial induction (medication)
- D&C

If your baby is *older* than about 12 weeks gestation (about the beginning of the second trimester), you may be given these options for delivery:

- artificial induction (medication)
- D&C
- D&E

You are invited to share your story here as well: please remember that sharing your story at stillbirthday is a way to express your feelings and share your experiences with other mothers – it is not to diagnose, treat or answer any medical questions.

You might visit our farewell celebrations for ideas to celebrate your baby.

COMPLETE MISCARRIAGE

This means that the baby has already been delivered, and the *entire* uterine lining and placenta have also been expelled.
This means that you are no longer pregnant.
If your pregnancy was very early, you can learn more about what happened from the natural miscarriage article.

Please visit these pages for additional support:

- Taking care of your emotional/spiritual health.
- You can still honor your baby, even if your miscarriage was some time ago. Please visit our farewell celebrations article for ideas.
- Please consider sharing your story with us.
- We also have a listing of long term support services.

LIVE MISCARRIAGE
OR, BORN ALIVE PRIOR TO VIABILITY

When a baby dies in the first 28 days of life after birth, it is called "neonatal death".

Because by most calculations a baby is considered viable in or after the 24th week of pregnancy, technically a stillborn baby who is born live, even for an extremely short time past delivery, may also be considered under the "neonatal death" category.

There is no such category for the unique situation in which a baby born via miscarriage either is or appears to be alive for seconds or even minutes after the birth.

Because there is no such technical category, but because parents who experience this unique and extremely special situation wish to have their baby's experiences validated, stillbirthday has identified this situation as "live miscarriage".

A live miscarriage may be most likely to occur the closer the baby is to reaching viability status (perhaps 16 weeks and older).

In a live miscarriage, immediately after the delivery, the baby may curl his or her fingers around the parents' finger, may either appear to take a breath (as air is pushed into his or her body, particularly when moved), or he or she may indeed take an actual breath.

Witnessing such movements or signs of life can either be alarming to parents, or, for others, can be extremely validating and profoundly significant.

For this reason, stillbirthday wishes to validate this rare but important experience by naming it "live miscarriage".

You won't know if your baby will display moments of signs of life, until after your experience is over and your baby is born. Please do not allow this to change the course of your birth plans, if your birth plans are medically necessary. Here are stories shared by mothers who've experienced a live miscarriage.

27

The following information continues to give you support through the miscarriage process:

If your baby is *younger* than about 12 weeks gestation, you may be given three options for delivery:
- natural delivery
- artificial induction (medication)
- D&C

If your baby is *older* than about 12 weeks gestation (about the beginning of the second trimester), you may be given these options for delivery:
- artificial induction (medication)
- D&C
- D&E

You are invited to share your story here as well: please remember that sharing your story at stillbirthday is a way to express your feelings and share your experiences with other mothers – it is not to diagnose, treat or answer any medical questions.

You might visit our farewell celebrations for ideas to celebrate your baby.

VANISHING TWIN OR PAPYRACEUS

"Vanishing Twin Syndrome" may occurs when a mother miscarries one of the twins she is pregnant with.

If the miscarriage happens *in the first trimester*, neither you nor your other baby should have any clinical signs or symptoms. The surviving twin usually still has an excellent probability of resulting in a full pregnancy and live birth, but it depends on the factors that contributed to the death of the other twin.

When a baby dies *after about eight weeks*, this baby and his or her placenta may likely be compressed from the pressure of the growth by the surviving twin; this is known as fetus papyraceus or papyrus. Generally, what is being compressed is the water that holds the small baby's soft structure while developing in the womb. Your doctor may inform you that your body has "reabsorbed" this water (or the baby), which might be *very* painful to hear. Because the baby's tiny tissues are no longer alive, your body may recognize your baby as a wound and begin to heal this wound by embracing the dead tissue to prevent it from further harming your body. You might consider something of like a scrape on your arm that your body scabs to heal. In this way, even your womb testifies to the painful experience you are going through.

It is possible that fetus papyraceus can occur in a singleton or a multiples pregnancy.

With twins, while both twins may be delivered, you should know what to expect to see if you want to be able to see the twin that has died (his or her physical form will likely be flattened and developmentally incomplete). If the twin died in the second or third trimester, there are increased risks to your other baby, including a possibility of having cerebral palsy and death. These risks depend on if the babies shared a placenta, or each had their own. For this

29

reason, your doctor may suggest artificially inducing your labor prior to reaching full term.

You can view a photo of twins, shared by a courageous stillbirthday mother, one born alive and the other who died via fetus papyraceus, here.

Your doctor will discuss with you the possible need to induce delivery of your twins, and the likelihood of this baby's survival. Please visit the specialized birth planning for giving birth to multiples (when one **or** both are still).

You are invited to share your story here as well: please remember that sharing your story at stillbirthday is a way to express your feelings and share your experiences with other mothers – it is not to diagnose, treat or answer any medical questions.

You might visit our farewell celebrations for ideas to celebrate your baby.

TWINS, MULTIPLES, HIGHER ORDER MULTIPLES

Also see our informational article on Vanishing Twin.

If you haven't done so already, please consider transferring your medical care to a Multiples Birth Specialist.

Please visit any of our specialized birth plans for giving birth to twins or multiples (when one or more are still) which also includes additional resources regarding multiples pregnancy. You might also visit our rainbow birth plan, as many mothers refer to their surviving multiple/s as rainbow babies.

Are you a mother who has endured a loss or losses involving a multiples pregnancy? Are you a surviving multiple? You are invited to share your story here .

You might visit our farewell celebrations for ideas to celebrate your baby or babies who are not alive.

SELECTIVE REDUCTION OR
TERMINATION FOR MEDICAL REASONS (TFMR)

Selective Reduction is a difficult decision families may face when pregnant with multiples. If one or more multiple potentially pose a danger to the health or wellbeing of the mother and/or siblings, the pressure to face this difficult decision may be even greater.
Because there are many different facets to such a difficult decision, we've divided them here to start with a general platform, simply to remind you that very fact – that there are many facets to such a difficult decision.

Regarding Loss after Medically Assisted Conception
- Loss after ART

Regarding Selective Reduction *specifically*
Here are external links to resources that are specific to selective reduction:
- In *Embracing Laura* , Martha Wegner-Hay tells her story of grief and joy after discovering she was pregnant with twins, that one twin would not survive, and giving birth to her healthy son, David. After being told that one of her twins had almost no chance of survival and that the sick baby could affect the chance of survival of the healthy twin, Wegner-Hay and her family made the difficult choice of selective reduction. *Embracing Laura* tells of the wrenching collision of sadness at Laura's death, and the joyous experience of David's healthy birth.
- Outside the Circle of Grief

Regarding Decisions & Loss
- In a deep desire to be sensitive, one of the facets of such a decision does include TFMR (termination for medical reasons), the intentional termination of life of one or more of

the babies, and so with this introduction to this facet you might visit our starting place for elective abortion as it does hold information that may be applied into the very specific situation of TFMR such as selective reduction as well.

Regarding NICU

- The NICU can be a difficult place to be in, emotionally, for any reason you may be there. Our NICU support resources are here to help.

Regarding Multiples

- Here is our start page regarding multiples, which links to additional outside resources for pregnancy challenges and support, birth plans and bereavement support.

ELECTIVE ABORTION

For every reason you may be here at this page, know this one thing: *you are loved.*

A Glimpse of Grief:

While this website provides support to mothers who are already enduring the actualized or inevitable death of their baby via pregnancy & infant loss, this article begins by serving mothers facing elective abortion, in hopes that if there truly is *any* choice whatsoever, you won't *have* to need the sort of grief support the rest of this website provides, because grief is real, it can be hard, and it can be a part of your story for the rest of your life. There can be tremendous hope, healing and joy in grief, but these things may not ever entirely fill the chasm.

When a baby dies for any reason, mothers may grieve for them. It is an ongoing process of healing. The grief that mothers who have experienced elective abortion face can become compounded by a guilt that mothers who have *not* faced a decision about the duration of life in-utero may not share (knowledgeisempowering.com). This intense struggle impacts many aspects of the mother's life: the post abortive mother may be at an increased risk for depression and physical health risks associated directly and indirectly with the elective abortion decision (afterabortion.org)

Loss After Deciding to Continue – *Were you at one point in your pregnancy vulnerable to considering elective abortion, determined to continue the pregnancy, and then endured an unexpected pregnancy loss? This particular experience can create complex feelings of guilt, shame and confusion. Consider this: in any fleeting moment during the elective abortion and birth processes, a mother may face intense regret, and a change of heart and mind that feels like the experience is robbing her completely. Please, be gentle on yourself.*

You can also visit our types of pregnancy loss list to get support specific to the type of loss and birth method you are experiencing, and consider sharing your story here, so that other mothers enduring this experience after you will find validation in their complex feelings of experiencing unexpected loss after determining to continue a vulnerable pregnancy.

Possible Pre-Abortion Support:

Here is a list of the most common reasons mothers may face an elective abortion decision, along with a few resources that may be of benefit to the challenges presented. Following these alternative resource options, there are support resources listed for you for the journey after facing this enormously complex, deeply vulnerable decision.

When you are faced with making a decision regarding the duration of life in-utero, any decision you make (parenting through elective abortion, adoption, or rearing), having had to face the decision itself can be excruciating and even traumatic. Reaffirming that you are intrinsically worthy of respect, dignity and love is vital.

You are worthy. You are worthy.

Challenges & Support:

"I just don't think I can parent."

Possible Options:

Our Birth & Bereavement Doulas can offer birth education, birth support, and early parenting preparation, including supplementing additional resources.

There are several different kinds of parenting resources available in every community, including free classes at hospitals, and library books on the topic.

The Baby Moses Project offers information and support options for parents who have tried to parent their child but through various circumstances, no longer feel capable of providing for their child.

In addition, put these terms in your search engine to get even more support from your location, including local crisis pregnancy centers.

"This pregnancy was from an affair, and I fear my marriage won't survive if my husband finds out."

Possible Options:

Whatever accountability issue there is surrounding this pregnancy, there are many resources to support you.

Whoever you are afraid of telling, there are professionals in your community ready to support you.

Crisis Pregnancy Centers may provide tips for your situation, as well as referrals to applicable sources.

Marriage counselors are availabe in every community, through independent listings, bookstore sections on marriage crises or through churches.

"I am young. I have my whole life ahead of me."

Possible Options:

Two things are important to know regarding making a decision to electively abort because you are young. One is that, there are many resources that serve to support you carrying your baby to term while assisting with finishing school and gaining employment. Second, it is important to know that elective abortion has serious long term consequences, and elective abortion performed on young women poses serious, *additional* risks (teenbreak.com).

You can call 1.800.395.4357

Text "TEEN" to 95495

24/7 online chat: option line

In addition, put these terms in your search engine to get even more support from your location.

"I can't afford to take care of this baby."

Possible Options:

Child Support

Government Assistance Programs

Local programs for single parents/low income

Credit card debt support

Mortgage/financial help

SPAOA

Continuing education financial support

In addition, put these terms in your search engine to get even more support from your location.

"I won't have a place to live if I keep this baby."

Possible Options:

Housing Assistance

SPAOA

HUD Housing / HUD.org

Apartments with special programs for single mothers

Pregnancy/mother shelters

Battered women shelters

Au Pair (pronounced "we pair")

In addition, put these terms in your search engine to get even more support from your location.

"My personal safety is in danger if I keep this baby."

Possible Options:

Elective abortion will not inherently increase your safety. If you are in an unsafe situation, it will continue to be unsafe whether you decide on elective abortion or not. You need to get into a safe situation, and there are many resources and places that serve to provide your safety, whichever decision you make regarding elective abortion.

Restraining orders/Ex Parte orders

Pregnancy/mother shelters

Battered and abused women shelters

In addition, put these terms in your search engine to get even more support from your location.

"Selective Reduction: I cannot parent all of these multiples."

Possible Options:

In a culture that has a shortsighted and lofty, almost magical idealism about the splendor of raising multiples, the truth is, raising multiples is enormously challenging. Coupled with the news that any of the multiples might be facing gestational or chromosomal abnormalities, a mother pregnant with multiples might be faced with the decision of what might be called *multifetal pregnancy reduction* or *selective reduction.*

Many of the same resources on this page might be applied in this situation as well.

Our multiples entry page links to practical information for such experiences as twinless twins, which also can be applied in this situation.

Multifetal Pregnancy Reduction, written by Jumelle

Embracing Laura

"The baby has something wrong with him."

Possible Options:

It is extremely important to get a second opinion, from a different hospital, before you make a decision regarding the duration of life in-utero.

Learn what the process of carrying to term is like.

Special Needs Adoption

There are resources that support mothers who are carrying to term babies with all kinds of diagnoses:

Alexandra's House offers, among other things, prenatal and postnatal housing

Madison's Foundation

Congenital Heart Support

String of Pearls

Congenital Diaphragmatic Hernia Support

Congenital Diaphragmatic Hernia Support

Congenital Diaphragmatic Hernia Support

Trisomy Support (13 or 18 or related)

Trisomy Support (13 or 18)

Trisomy 18 support

Trisomy 13 support

Anencephaly support

Prader-Willi Syndrome Support

Spina Bifida Support

Cleft Lip/Palate Support (and related)

Prenatal Partners for Life

Be Not Afraid

Sufficient Grace

Waiting with Love

Beads of Courage

Project Sunshine

NICU support/micropreemie/preemie (scroll to bottom)

Noah's Dad – raising a child with Down's Syndrome from a dad's perspective

These are only a very small number of resources. Please, go slow. You are worthy of support for every single part of this experience you are facing.

In addition, put these terms in your search engine to get even more support from your location.

"No, really. My baby is going to die. It's literally just a matter of when."

Possible Options:

It is extremely important to get a second opinion, from a different hospital, before you make a decision regarding the duration of life in-utero.

Learn what the process of carrying to term is like.

There can be physical, hormonal, emotional, spiritual and psychological benefits to carrying to term. However, carrying to term (or, waiting for spontaneous onset of labor) can also pose very real psychospiritual, social and relational challenges that need to be addressed. Weighing these decisions is an impossible time. What mainstream religious or political agendas don't share openly is that when the death of your baby is entirely unavoidable, as in a diagnosed and confirmed fatal diagnosis, there can be some sense of empowerment in a situation that feels so entirely out of your control, in making such decisions as scheduling the medically assisted birth of your baby, while so doing, forfeiting any or all medicalized life sustaining or death delaying treatment. In a situation such as this, when all circumstances except the date of death and birth are out of your control, the term "elective abortion" may be especially triggering or feel insensitive. The sense of empowerment though, in setting an induction date, can be ongoing, or, it can be fleeting and be met with long term regret. Each member of your care team should be aware and extremely honoring to this truth. "Making a decision and sticking with it" isn't really a reasonable expectation. More in line with the enormity of such a time is to give yourself permission to experience your feelings, and to treat yourself with love. None of this is easy. In any and all of your decisions, go slow. It may feel impossible to go slow, but you can, and prepare your resources for your journey ahead.

"My doctor told me I could die if I don't terminate the pregnancy."

Possible Options:

Like all diagnosis situations, getting a second opinion is always in your best interest.

If your baby has a fatal condition, and waiting for the baby to die naturally poses danger to your own life, here is information particular to your unique situation.

We also have support and resources for children and loved ones when there has been Maternal Death.

Post Elective Abortion

You have Dignity, Worth, and Love

If you have come to this site and have faced elective abortion at any time in the past, seeing the many different perspectives and alternatives, can re-open your wounds and place that heavy burden of guilt on your heart all over again. Grief after elective abortion can look different for each mother. In your grief, you might experience any feelings that are universal to bereaved mothers, such as longing, sadness, or anger. You might also experience feelings of relief, or even feelings of *guilt* at feeling relief. Still other mothers believe that the feelings of regret or shame they may experience are deserved, as if enduring a life of humiliation and comdemnation allows them to bear pain they wanted to protect their children from. These are all complex emotions, and each of them deserve to be looked at lovingly, with a goal of holistic healing. Please know that *you are not alone*, and that there are resources to help you heal, from immediately postpartum, to the lifelong healing journey ahead. Stillbirthday is designed to bring light into the chasm. We are all in this together.

I am Sorry

In some situations, a mother who has decided upon elective abortion may not identify this decision with a "loss". You may not feel a baby died. Your own personal convictions may be that your situation was the "potential" for life, or, that your baby may return to you in a future pregnancy. Into these beliefs, telling you that I am sorry for your loss may not quite fit. But even still, elective abortion can have a substantial print upon your impression of your body image, your feminine identity and your journey. The flow of grief may bring in the occasional shift of breeze that has new questions or new feelings. All of your experiences and all of your feelings are worthy to be looked at with recognition and love. Whatever situation itself that perhaps wasn't the most fertile ground for alternatives to elective abortion, may have been itself a kind of loss, a situation that may hold pain or grief to you. Incest. An unstable relationship. Pressures that made the decision for you. In a later season in which some of these things may change, once again those breezes may blow past your heart and bring fresh questions and feelings. I am sorry. Because being a woman comes with more responsibility than we are ever taught in high school. Because learning to love ourselves is a higher calling than any religious message credits it for. Because we holders of wombs can rip each other to shreds to substantiate our own merit. I am sorry, because I too do not always get things right. I am sorry that it took such a painful subject for us to be real with one another, even here in a tiny written paragraph. I will not wait any longer to tell you. No matter what, you are loved.

Subsequent Pregnancy

Particularly the first pregnancy after elective abortion, you may face the feelings any mother pregnant after loss may endure. In addition to things like climactic milestones in pregnancy (reaching the point in pregnancy in which a diagnosis was determined in a previous pregnancy, the gestational week of birth, or other important points to you), you may find that there are physical and emotional reactions to this pregnancy. The method of medicalized birth, for example, can bring with it long term consequences, such as scarring or impact on fertility and subsequent miscarriage. Emotionally, the pregnancy or climactic milestones within it may be met with fresh grief, fear, guilt, shame, and you may experience stretches of emotional dystocia in labor (a physical delay prompted in part or entirety by emotional implications). However, the emotional impact of a subsequent pregnancy, birth, and choosing an adoption plan or a parenting-through-rearing plan may bring a particular sense of affirmation, reconciliation, peace, and joy. Any or all of these experiences or reactions can be a healthy part of your journey. The decision you have faced regarding the duration of life in-utero is only one part of your story – an important part, but only one part. You can consider how you might define your experience and the unique ways in which you might approach the multitude of aspects of your journey. Maybe you don't feel comfortable sharing openly that you have faced a decision, but, in a subsequent pregnancy, birth or welcoming, you might want to incorporate "rainbows" – which is a common sign among bereaved mothers who have endured pregnancy and infant loss who have a subsequent pregnancy or living baby. Whatever you decide, is as unique and beautiful as you. Please visit our Getting Pregnant Again resources for mothers pregnant after enduring pregnancy and infant loss.

Healing Resources:

SBD Farewell Celebrations

stories contributed by mothers

1.877.586.4621 (Lumina)

1.866.4.EXHALE

National Memorial for the Unborn

Exhale

Hope After Abortion

Post Abortive Reconciliation

After Abortion.org

Your Backline

Bethesda

Lumina

ARIN (Abortion Recovery InterNational)

Rachel's Vineyard (Q&A, retreats, stories)

Supportive Book Listing

Infant Loss Blog Directory has a listing of medical termination blogs (scroll down on the right)

In recognition of the 40th anniversary of Roe v. Wade, CNN published hundreds of small video clips from mothers who have faced elective abortion.

In addition, put these terms in your search engine to get even more support from your location.

You are also invited to share your story with us.

All Are Welcome Here (Please do not drop your flowers and run. You are loved.)

RECURRENT MISCARRIAGE
OR FERTILITY STRUGGLE

This article contains general information regarding recurrent miscarriage, stillbirth, and fertility information. If you are miscarrying right now, please be taken back to the beginning for immediate miscarriage support.

Enduring multiple losses can pose unique emotional challenges, whether you have surviving children or not, and whether you have surviving children or not, emotional support is extremely important. Having a surviving child or children can make you feel as though your feelings over your losses are perhaps less valuable, and well-meaning friends can inflict unintentional harm as they pry and ask questions about your continued family planning, not knowing you may be enduring such heartbreak. If you do not have surviving children, the journey from grief to healing can seem excruciatingly lonely, hopeless, and as though noone could understand your many feelings, including how to handle family pressures to carry on the family name or legacy, or planning your retirement years without children or grandchildren involved.

Whether a few weeks, or a few years, have passed since your first pregnancy loss, any subsequent losses are usually more emotionally devastating on both the mother and the father, and the intensity of the grief can oftentimes seem magnified.

Following subsequent losses, it can seem as though you may be trying to numb or dull the emotions out.

You may have at one time processed your feelings and felt confident that if you experience another loss, you may be more ready, more in control. Oftentimes, it is one parent who feels this confidence, while the other parent may have doubts or fears about trying again. You may feel guilty or embarrassed for thinking you could try again, or for thinking that you could handle another loss easier. You may feel so angry that you decide to make a definitive decision regarding birth control, or you may feel so panicked that you quickly try again. You may wonder why it is so unfair that you have recurrent losses, and may wonder if you'll ever complete a full pregnancy with a happy, healthy baby. You may feel that after subsequent losses, it is best to be quiet about it, not tell anyone, and try to move on silently.

These feelings are all very common, and you really can work through them positively.

And, you are not alone. Please consider sharing your story with us, so that another mother experiencing recurrent pregnancy loss can learn from you.

There are all kinds of support resources here at stillbirthday, from immediate support through the process of loss, to later, long term support resources.

Here are links to several different ideas and sources of information (outside links) that you might find useful. Please discard any resource that does not find comfort in your heart. This is not a place of imposing anyone's position onto you in your journey, or even of endorsing any resource, but simply of presenting different opportunities for you. It is my deepeset desire that you can find a way, a person, or a place, that you feel comfortable talking about your feelings and getting the support that you need.

Multiple pregnancy loss is devastating, and emotional healing is extremely important. Please, as you grieve, and find your way to healing, be gentle with yourself.

Stillbirthday Additional Links:

threatened miscarriage (and some tips)

facts/stats on pregnancy & infant loss

getting pregnant again

loss after medically assisted conception (or ART)

ending fertility in loss

farewell celebrations

Perspectives from Other Mothers:

The Pregnancy Companion (on fertility, adoption, and more)

My Yellow Brick Road Has Potholes

Operation Heads Up (on fertility options)

Peer Infertility Counselors

Professional Fertility Support / Referrals

Fertile Heart

Fertility LifeLine

Prayers for Conception:

Hannah's Tears

Productive Two Week Wait

Sarah's Laughter

Identifying Primary Infertility:

Resolve

A TIME (Jewish support)

Identifying Secondary Infertility:

Resolve

Important Aspects and Links to Fertility Challenges:

Facts/Stats

Fertility after Cancer

Non-Medical Fertility Support:

Fertile Heart

Our Cultural Keepsakes section might be valuable to you.

As with anything, remember to consult your medical care provider.

Non-Medical Fertility and Healthy Links:

Parenting Begins Before Conception

Birth Art Cafe

Pre-Conception Tea

N0n-Traditional Family Support Resources:

Family Creation Network

Medically Assisted Conception:

Ovulation Induction

Ovarian Drilling

Intrauterine Insemination

Female Surgery: Laparoscopy

Female Surgery: Tubal Sterilization Reversal

Female Surgery: Hydrosalpinx Removal

Male Surgery: Testicular Biopsy

Male Surgery: Testicular Sperm Aspiration (TESA)

Male Surgery: Percutaneus Sperm Aspiration (PESA)

In Vitro Fertilization (IVF)

Embryo Donation and Adoption

Embryo Adoption Awareness

Blastocyst/Embryo Transfer

Traditional Surrogacy / Gestational Surrogacy

Surrogacy Laws by State

"All Things Surrogacy"

Foster/Adoption:

Foster/Adopt State-by-State Directory

Adoption Agency Ratings

Center for Adoption Support and Education

Adoption Questions

Missing Grace Foundation

Adoption Doulas or any of our SBD Doulas

Finding Peace with Childlessness:

Beside the Empty Cradle (website)

Beside the Empty Cradle (book)

NICU GRIEF

We have information specific to difficult and fatal diagnosis, including a large listing of outside resources. Please visit our birth plan that can link you to carrying to term information in addition to these outside links specific to diagnoses.

If your baby has received a diagnosis or is expected to receive care in the NICU, here is a list of resources. Please continue to the end of this article for information about *the reality of NICU grief.*

Information for Your Loved Ones:

NICU/Special Needs & Loved Ones

Prenatal Educational & Emotional Support:

Prenatal Process & Support (both surviving & fatal diagnosis)

Bliss

Immediate & Long Term Informational & Practical Support Resources for Surviving Diagnosis:

Infant Disability Resources by State (this large library collection includes a *long term parenting list of resources*)

NICU Items:

Books & Websites relating to the process of carrying to term with a fatal diagnosis

NICU specific clothing

NICU/micropreemie diapers

NICU photography

NICU Support:

Graham's Foundation

Zoe's New Beginnings

Project Sweet Peas

NICU Research & Information:

Some providers discourage parents from touching extreme preemie babies receiving NICU care. This article can give more information on why that is, and what you may be able to do.

Get Connected:

Share your story here.

Join our blogroll and other writings here.

Faith's Lodge & Stillbirthday Mothers Workshops

Many of these are web links that are added to and updated regularly online, but which can't be used through your text, so please visit www.stillbirthday.com for support.

NEONATAL DEATH

When a baby dies in the first 28 days of life, it is technically called a neonatal death.

I personally find technical timeframes like this to be arbitrary in our emotional interpretation of our experiences, and I hardly think the term addresses the enormous amount of feeling we may have. We do at stillbirthday provide support for every technical name, medical label, and timeframe category of parental bereavement, including all of the many names for pregnancy loss, neonatal death, older infancy, and toddlers to teens. Just visit here to learn more.

Some parents know ahead of time that their preborn baby may have a condition "not compatible with life" after birth. While these parents may in some ways prepare for the birth of their baby and try to anticipate the very short time they may have with their baby, the experiences are heartwrenching, agonizing and painful.

For these parents, already having a personalized birth plan may help support them through the process.

Still other parents go on to deliver a healthy child, and without any notice or warning whatsoever, the child dies.

In either case, this website offers a number of supportive services:

information regarding the process from realization to farewell celebration (including a customized birth plan for no or short expectancy of life, and another to serve families when given extra time, and additional resources for various diagnoses). The PROCESS link is extremely valuable.

statistics

information for friends and family on how to best support you professionals and volunteers to support you

local, national, and international long-term support services and resources including books

farewell celebration ideas

a place to share your story

a place to read a story or two from other parents and see their babies photos

please visit our Love Cupboard for newborn clothing support which may prove useful when given extra time.

BIRTH METHODS

The way your baby will be born.

Birth methods include the recommended ways, techniques and tools involved to provide the safest birth experience for you.

METHOTREXATE

Methotrexate is administered to mothers who have been diagnosed with an ectopic pregnancy very early in their pregnancy (generally about 6 weeks and under). It can be given orally, however, it is usually recommended that it be administered by injection, with either one or two injection sites. It is considered a noninvasive procedure and reduces the amount of scarring to your reproductive organs. On rare occasions, this medication may also be administered *after* laparoscopic surgery to prevent any cells from growing that may have been left behind.

The medication will simply tell your baby to stop working.

After the medication is administered, you will probably be allowed to return home, with a follow up appointment a few days to a week later.

Within that time, your baby's efforts to grow will be rested to the point that the baby dies.

You will bleed just as in a natural miscarriage, for at least the first few days.

You can make this birth method more meaningful by incorporating your own birth plan.

How far along are you? Because ectopic pregnancy can be fatal to the mother unless the pregnancy ends as quickly as possible, I will only include very early development links to fetal information (and there is a probability that the development of an ectopic baby may be a little different; still, it can be nice to have a general idea of what your baby's last developments will be):

4 weeks

5 weeks

6 weeks

Your doctor will advise you against using any of the following, as they can interfere with the concentration of medication:

vitamins containing folic acid (including prenatal vitamins)

alcohol

penicillin

ibuprofen

Your doctor will also cover side effects and warning signs with you, including discussing the potential risks Methotrexate (possibly referred to as chemotherapy) can have on trying to conceive in the near future. Some studies indicate that the medicine from Methotrexate may remain present in your own body's cells for up to 7 months after use; doctors generally recommend waiting at least one ovulation cycle before TTC after Methotrexate to prevent complications in fetal growth in the subsequent pregnancy.

LAPAROSCOPIC BIRTH

Surgery for ectopic pregnancy may either be laparoscopy (explained here) or minilaparotomy.

Because ectopic pregnancy can be fatal to the mother unless the pregnancy ends as quickly as possible, I will only include very early development links to fetal information (and there is a probability that the development of an ectopic baby may be a little different; still, it can be nice to have a general idea of what your baby's last developments will be). This surgical birth method may be used if methotrexate was ineffective.

The full medical term for laparoscopic surgery is "Laparascopic Salpingotomy". Laparoscopic surgery is performed under general anesthesia. Your doctor will use a tool called a laparoscope to enter your abdomen through a small incision, deliver the baby, and to repair any affected part of the fallopian tube.

Once the doctor determines the condition of the fallopian tube, if it is not repairable, a "Laparoscopic Salpingectomy" will be performed (a "laparotomy", which is a larger abdominal incision, may be required), which is the partial or the complete removal of the damaged fallopian tube.

You can make this birth method more meaningful by incorporating your own birth plan.

Development:

- 4 weeks
- 5 weeks
- 6 weeks
- 7 weeks
- 8 weeks

"NATURAL" MISCARRIAGE

Natural miscarriage means waiting for the miscarriage to complete on its own. A benefit to miscarrying naturally is knowing for certain that your baby in fact has died (see concerns with D&C). It also allows you to spend time gathering your feelings and processing the transition from experiencing hopes and joy to experiencing loss. A common concern that your medical provider may have about you miscarrying naturally, is is the risk of postpartum hemorrhage. The risk of complications of a natural miscarriage is increased, the older the baby was when he or she died. Generally, studies indicate that approximately 70% of mothers who miscarry naturally do so without unexpected complications. Natural miscarriage is safest if the baby's gestational age is younger than *10 weeks*. If you and your medical provider have both determined that natural miscarriage would be a safe option for you, it is important to know what to expect and how to prepare yourself.

If at any time you fill a maxi pad sooner than a half hour, experience dizziness, tingling in your hands or feet, or a racing heart (or any of these even with light bleeding), you should consult a medical professional immediately.

INDUCTION/AUGMENTATION

Medication can help stimulate labor, and allow you to birth your baby.

These are a few common medications that are used to help deliver miscarried babies, and they may be given separately or in conjunction with each other:

- mifepristone
- misoprostol
- methylergometrine (methergine)

Mifepristone blocks a hormone (progesterone) from completing its pregnancy function of supporting the uterine lining that the baby has been growing in. This will stop your body's efforts of sustaining the pregnancy. In some cases, this will be enough to trigger "permission" to your body to begin expelling the placenta and delivering your baby.

Misoprostol (a prostaglandin) causes your uterus to contract, so that your baby can be delivered. "Cytotec" is one prescription name used, and misoprostol is said to have about an 80-90% effectiveness rate in delivering miscarried babies and completely expelling all of the placenta pieces.

Methergine helps to control excessive bleeding and can cause your uterus to contract, so that your baby can be delivered.

You may be asked to stay at the hospital to deliver your baby, or you may be permitted to deliver your baby at home. This will depend on the age of your baby, and other factors including your hospital's policies.

Using labor stimulating medication to help with the delivery of your baby in early pregnancy is generally considered a medically safe approach, one that doesn't have the possible adverse side effects as more medically involved births. In rare instances, medication does not deliver the entire placenta, and more medically assisted support (D&C) may be needed to help completely deliver the placenta. When using a labor stimulant to help in the delivery of a very young baby, you should expect to see a heavier blood discharge than your menstrual period, and possibly small tissue-like pieces of uterine lining. Your baby's placenta, as it detaches from your uterine wall, is very soft and will most likely break into smaller pieces. By the eighth week of pregnancy, the placenta is about the size of a peach, and by the twelfth week it's about the size of a pear, and so the pieces as it is delivered may roughly be the size of grapes.

Your doctor will discuss with you the side effects and warning signs to look out for when taking induction medication, including fever, too much bleeding (hemorrhage), and the amount of time it should take to complete the entire process.

Generally, you will probably be cautioned that filling a regular-absorbancy maxi pad sooner than one hour, at any time, is cause of concern; immediately postpartum (that is, right after the baby is born), generally speaking you should not fill a regular-absorbancy maxi pad sooner than a half-hour in the first hour (so, you can go through 2 pads in the first hour postpartum), as it is common to experience some increased bleeding at the actual time of delivery. Besides medication to help stimulate labor, other options to assist in the dilation of your cervix may include **seaweed laminaria** or the use of a **Foley catheter**. The Foley catheter (sometimes called Foley ball or bulb) will manually dilate your cervix; this is not a medication but is instead a tool/instrument. Your doctor will insert the Foley into your vagina and the process can be uncomfortable but should resemble a vaginal exam. The ball has a small tube at the end of it. After the ball is in place, the doctor will fill up the ball like a balloon. The sensations from the Foley vary to feeling bloated, crampy, to a feeling of having tetanic (constant) contractions. As you dilate large enough, the Foley will fall out. Each of these options can help dilate your cervix to approximately 3 or 4 centimeters, which should be enough for early pregnancy loss. Pregnancy losses that occur later in pregnancy may be supplemented by the use of Pitocin to continue to dilate the cervix for birth.

Your doctor will discuss these options with you according to your unique situation.

If at any time you fill a maxi pad sooner than a half hour, experience dizziness, tingling in your hands or feet, or a racing heart (or any of these even with light bleeding), you should consult a medical professional immediately.

If you are hoping to be able to find and identify your baby, the chances are increased if you have a general understanding of what to expect to find. The following links will take you to information on the stages of development and the size of the baby.

LEVELS OF AUGMENTATION

There are various ways to help facilitate some change in the progress of labor. Many are listed here, in order from least interventive ("natural") to more interventive ("medical"). Please know that many "natural" techniques are not scientifically proven and/or their effectiveness may be in conjunction with dangerous side effects. Please discuss all "natural" options with your care provider (OB or midwife), whether or not your doula is versed on the topic or not, including exactly how to prepare or present the option. We also note in our early at-home birth plan, that it is possible to experience what we refer to here at stillbirthday as "early pregnancy prodromal labor" – your labor may or may not start and stop, unexpectedly. It is also, enormously important for you to know, for your emotional well being, that even if a "natural" option *might* help in the augmentation of labor, *this does not mean that it caused your loss.* These options are listed here because it has been noted by other mothers, that *once the birthing process has already begun,* these options have been reported by them as being in some way helpful.

Please utilize any of the many emotional support resources we have available at stillbirthday.

External

- walking, lunging, singing, praying/meditating (entering into a safe physical place to do so), relaxing, car ride, oxytocin release (doula can support), massage, effleurage, brushing teeth, hydrotherapy, various "yoga" type positions (doula can support), chiropractic care, herbal bath: yarrow, sage, oregano and nettle.
- stillbirthday has a proprietary collection of healing essential oils, but *shipment times need to be considered.*

External – More Intensive

- nipple stimulation, accupressure/puncture

Internal

- raspberry leaf tea, Lady's Mantle, wine of ergot (spurred rye), eggplant parmesan, oregano, pineapples, spicy foods, "labor cookies", intercourse, coffee or other stimulants
- Spatone, chlorophyll, Floradix, hemoplex, spirulina, alfalfa, red clover or nettle can help restore iron drained through blood loss.
- deep reflection into possibilities of emotional dystocia: prayer, meditation, reflection, permission to heal

Internal – More Intensive

- cohoshes, primrose, fresh parsley, castor oil/enema, cotton root bark, angelica, pennyroyal (please see this external article regarding herbal augmentation) , vodka (some believe that any alcohol, however, can actually stall labor. Again, all of these *need* to be discussed with your provider.)

Medical

- vaginal exams, stripping membranes, cervical ripening agents (Misoprostil), Foley bulb (see Artificial Induction birth method for information on Misoprostil, Foley and other augmentation options)

Medical – More Intensive

- Cytotec, Pitocin, forceps/vacuum/episiotomy, or planned or emergency Cesarean Birth(see Full Term Birth Plan for information on these options)

EARLY TO MID PREGNANCY MEDICALLY ASSISTED BIRTH

D&C AND D&E

If your doctor has recommended a D&E to help deliver your baby, the very first thing to consider is changing the perspective you may have about this approach.

Many mothers have very strong objections to having a D&E performed because of the comparison to an elective abortion.

A D&E is a way to medically assist in the delivery of a baby. The medical operation is the same if the baby is alive or not. But, the operation itself is not abortion. It is a medical way to assist in the delivery of your baby. If this method is needed, perhaps it might be more healing for you to consider it more of a **"vaginal Cesarean"**, in that the doctor is going to manually assist in the delivery of your tiny baby.

Another thing you may consider, is that some women recall feeling doubt or uncertainty that their child had in fact died prior to the D&E. This doubt is part of the grieving process, and is normal. But it can be terribly difficult to move past any feelings of doubt or uncertainty *after* the D&E has been performed. For this reason, I strongly suggest utilizing any ultrasound or doppler device that you can prior to the D&E. Perhaps contact a local *crisis pregnancy center* to see if they offer free ultrasounds. This extra step can provide you with the certainty you need in knowing that you are not "electively aborting" your baby. Remember, a D&E does *not* mean elective abortion.

The third thing to consider, is asking your provider if artificial induction may be a simpler, safer way to deliver your baby. Sometimes, a doctor will plan for a D&E (or a D&C, which is a different birth method that may also be an option to ask about) simply because it can be easier on you than trying to really navigate different approaches. Even if your doctor has recommended a D&E, it might be a good idea to just mention the option of artificial induction, and allow your provider to discuss your options with you so that you can have the safest delivery of your baby possible.

Now, with all of that said, a D &E (sometimes mistakenly called a DNE) is a method of delivery, used most often in *inevitable* or *missed* miscarriages, or for miscarriages that occur later in the second trimester, after your baby's bones have begun to harden (approximately at 16 weeks or older). It may also be used if a miscarriage had not completed naturally (any placenta fragments remain in the uterus). It is a combination of the D&C birth method, with additional delivery tools used, such as forceps, to help deliver your baby. We include additional information regarding this in our birth plan, where you might consider what questions or options you may have and create a dialogue with your trusted care provider about ways to learn the gender of your baby, physical characteristics, or anything else that might be of emotional value to you.

You may be given an antibiotic and/or pain medication, and physical recovery may include spotting for several days. Your birth plan for this method will include additional information. Generally, it is best to not plan on conceiving again until after you have had the first subsequent menstrual cycle, to ensure that your uterus is completely clear; waiting at least a week to introduce anything into your vagina (tampons, intercourse) is also recommended. Your provider will discuss these things with you. **You can make this birth method more meaningful by incorporating your own** birth plan.

ENCOURAGEMENT FOR BIRTH

These quotes and verses serve to bring encouragement to you *as you prepare for the birth of your baby.* Because pregnancy loss is still birth, these affirmations and encouragements are borrowed from childbirth websites (sources at end) and in fact are more fitting here than anywhere else.

As for you, be strong and courageous, for your work will be rewarded. ~ 2 Chronicles 15:7

"If I don't know my options, I don't have any." ~ Diana Korte

God arms me with strength, and he makes my way perfect. ~ Psalm 18:32

"There is a secret in our culture, and it's not that birth is painful. It's that women are strong." ~ Laura Stavoe Harm

The Lord will fight for you... ~Exodus 14:14a

"It seems that many health professionals involved in antenatal care have not realized that one of their roles should be to *protect the emotional state of pregnant women.*" ~Michel Odent, M.D.

God is our refuge and strength, an ever present help in time of trouble. ~ Psalm 46:1

"The effort to separate the physical experience of childbirth from the mental, emotional and spiritual aspects of this event has served to disempower and violate women." ~Mary Rucklos Hampton

The Lord your God is with you wherever you go. ~Joshua 1:9

"Fear can be overcome only by Faith." ~Grantly Dick-Read, M.D.

Though he brings grief, he will show compassion, so great is his unfailing love. ~Lamentations 3:44

Verses borrowed from: Scriptures for Childbirth
Quotes borrowed from: Birth Without Fear

BIRTH & BEREAVEMENT QUOTES

I would not undo his existence just to undo my pain. ~Stillbirthday Mother

Every baby is born. ~Cathy Gordon, CNM

Miscarriages are labor, miscarriages are birth. To consider them less dishonors the woman whose womb has held life, however briefly. ~ Kathryn Miller Ridiman

Sometimes the heart sees what is invisible to the eye. ~ H. Jackson Brown, Jr.

The love and bond between a mother and her child begins the very moment she knows they are on their way to her. ~ Vicki Reece

Waiting is painful. Forgetting is painful. But not knowing which to do is the worse kind of suffering. ~ Paulo Coelho

Hope is important because it can make the present moment less difficult to bear. If we believe that tomorrow will be better, we can bear a hardship today. ~ Thich Nhat Hanh

A very small degree of hope is sufficient to cause the birth of love. ~ Stendhal

I honor you. {I DO}ula. ~stillbirthday doula

A pregnancy loss is still a birthday.

MY WORDS

_____
_____
_____
_____
_____
_____
_____
_____
_____
_____
_____
_____

BIRTH PREPARATION
"BIRTH PLANS"

EARLY PREGNANCY HOME BIRTH

Things to know:
- You should *not* miscarry your baby at home alone.

Helpful tips:
- Check out our listing of local professionals and volunteers willing to support you through the process
- Consider special farewell words or music.
- Also include a personalized farewell celebration.
- Ask for your ultrasound photos, if any, or visit a local Crisis Pregnancy Center that performs ultrasounds, and ask if you can have one last photo of your baby.
- If your baby still has a heartbeat, consider using your cell phone or other recordable device, and record the doppler's sounds of your baby's heartbeat. You can then add this to a Build-A-Bear as a momento.
- More momento and special ideas are listed in the birth plan.
- If after the birth, you experience pain, fever, bleeding that fills a pad sooner than an hour, clotting, or a foul odor, please see your care provider immediately. Please view the article on postpartum hemorrhage.
- Our birth education section has additional information that may prove useful to you, including our Levels of Augmentation article that provides ways of naturally augmenting/speeding up the labor process.
- Please visit our link on general postpartum health (your emotional and physical health after delivery).

How far along are you? Do you know what to expect to possibly see? You are invited to view photos shared by other mothers.

For babies about 10-19 gestational weeks

Things to Have

Labor

__support person!

__phone (to call 911 if necessary)

__heavy maxi pads (no tampons)

__camera

__plenty of water to stay hydrated

__music and other soothing birth items and options, like massage, affirmations

__do not use a douche or enema to help labor progress

__several large old towels to catch blood in the birth space, especially around toilet

__ small fish net (or plastic bowl, colander, ladle or cheesecloth – you can rest the colander inside the toilet) to help screen or scoop from toilet

__latex gloves (dish or medical gloves) to help scoop from toilet

The Welcoming

__large sheet of tinfoil (or plastic wrap or wax paper) as a stable place to view your baby after birth __saline (contact solution) to use with clear cup

__clear shot glass or small vase (with saline solution: this helps restore your baby's fullness and can magnify his or her shape so you can see him or her more clearly)

__tweezers or toothpicks to help move fragmented pieces of placenta or sac without sticking and causing unnecessary ripping/sticking

Preparing for The Farewell

__if you are planning on bringing everything that you deliver to the hospital, including as much of the placenta as you can, you will need a large, gallon sized ziplock baggie (and a non-see through grocery sack or bag to place that in)

__special jewelry box or other special box for a coffin for your baby to be placed in

__a small square of pretty gift tissue with a little note that you can flush, or incorporating water in another way, particularly if flushing is inevitable

__be prepared for a possible ER visit

Things to do Before the Birth (while laboring)

__set up your bathroom and/or another room as the birth space. Fold edges of foil to make a large tray, and place this on your counter.

__call friends and family for support.

Things to Expect

__Sometimes bleeding will begin, and then completely stop (for hours or even days) before resuming.

__bleeding should not fill a heavy maxi pad sooner than one hour at any time during the labor.

__the placenta is between the size of a pear to a grapefruit, and will probably be expelled in grape sized pieces.

__very small, fleshy, flaky pieces of discharge are probably pieces of your uterine lining.

__every time you use the restroom, once bleeding has begun, you may expel pieces of placenta.

__it is easier to retrieve everything that is being expelled, to look through and identify your baby, if you hold the small fish net or colander underneath your vagina in the toilet bowl, than it is to allow everything to first be caught in the toilet and attempt to retrieve it after (because everything may be slippery)

__labor will likely peak right before the birth of your baby, at which time, for the first hour postpartum, bleeding may increase, but you should not fill a heavy maxi pad sooner than a half hour, during the first hour (after the first hour, bleeding should begin to taper off).

__know that your baby may not be born intact. He or she may physically be very unrecognizable.

__if you baby is born in his or her amniotic sac, he or she may appear to look very similar to the pieces of expelled placenta.

__when your baby is born, place him or her on the foil tray you have set up on your bathroom counter. Using the tweezers and foil creates a place you can gently pull back some of the additional sac fragments to simply look upon the physical form of your baby. Because physical changes happen rapidly, placing your baby into the clear jar of saline water can help draw out the fullness of his form again and continue to preserve him. You'll need to change this water at least every 4 hours if you choose to keep him in here longer.

__don't use toilet paper or Q tips to dry baby, as it may stick and pull at your baby's delicate skin. Instead, use tweezers, a toothpick, or your finger, and very gently move your baby away from the small puddle of blood, until he or she is more dry. Know that your baby will lose his shape very quickly after birth.

__Utilize all of the special plans you have, including saving mementos, holding your baby.

__name your baby, take photographs

__when you are ready, place your baby in the small Tupperware container and then in the special box.

__invite a spiritual advisor/leader and friends and family to join you after the baby is born (please consider though, that they may not choose to see your baby). See the "Professionals/Volunteers" link at stillbirthday.com for additional services to consider.

After the Birth

If you leave to the ER

__bring a fresh change of clothes with you.

__Have the photo you brought placed with your baby.

__Ask if baby can be swaddled in the blanket you brought (or just leave the blanket there)

__ask if you will be able to take your baby home with you, or if you can have your baby returned to you after any genetic testing is done.

At Home

__Have someone planning on spending the night with you. Perhaps consider having a friend spend the night with you, so that your husband can go home, prepare the house, and rest.

__You will still have lochia (the remaining blood from inside the uterus, which may be shed for the next 1-3 weeks).

__Watch for signs of postpartum depression (PPD) or secondary vaginitus.

__Be easy on yourself, your body, and on your recovery.

__Talk to your trusted spiritual advisors, your husband, and trusted mentors and friends about all of your feelings.

__*Visit stillbirthday.com for "Farewell Celebrations" and for "Long Term Support" resources.

Babies about 4-10 gestational weeks

Things to Have

    __The same supplies as listed above

Things to Expect

__labor (bleeding) should begin within two weeks of the death of your baby, but could take longer. Natural induction could include drinking raspberry tea.

__it will be very unlikely that you will be able to identify or retrieve your very tiny baby (flushing is very likely inevitable)

__name your baby

__include a trusted spiritual advisor and friends and family if you wish. See the "Professionals/Volunteers" link at stillbirthday.com for additional services to consider.

After the Birth

If you leave to the ER

__bring a fresh change of clothes with you.

__Have a photo you brought placed with your baby.

__Have a blanket or other special item left with your baby.

__ask if you will be able to take your baby home with you, or if you can have your baby returned to you after any genetic testing is done.

__bring a teddy bear or other item that you can hold on the car ride home.

At Home

__Have someone planning on spending the night with you. Perhaps consider having a friend spend the night with you, so that your husband can go home, prepare the house, and rest.

__You will still have lochia (the remaining blood from inside the uterus, which may be shed for the next 1-3 weeks).

__Watch for signs of postpartum depression (PPD) or secondary vaginitus.

__Be easy on yourself, your body, and on your recovery.

__Incorporate your spiritual beliefs, your husband, and trusted mentors and friends about all of your feelings.

__*Visit stillbirthday.com for "Farewell Celebrations" and for "Long Term Support" resources.

www.stillbirthday.com

EARLY PREGNANCY OPERATIVE BIRTH

**This plan is specific to early pregnancy (under 20 weeks) medicalized, operative birth.
Note that different aspects of the delivery will be different for the different gestational ages.**

Birth in hospital: you may be placed under general anesthesia, or sedation, and after the birth, you will stay in recovery for a few hours, when you will be discharged.

Birth at office : the doctor may administer local anesthesia, and your discharge will be in less than an hour (like a pelvic exam).

Please visit the previous chapter to become familiar with the ways in which stillbirthday offers a compassionate explanation and definition for the experience of a medically assisted birth in early or mid pregnancy.

During Birth

What to Bring

__camera

__someone to support you (to wait in waiting room, and to drive you home)

__additional support people can include a friend or chaplain

__photo of you and your husband to keep with baby

__Clinging Cross or something special to hold

__scented eye mask to wear during the birth

__*additional special items: two teddy bears or blankets (one to leave with your baby, and one to take home)

__Music and player (headphones) or battery operated personal fan, if permitted (to muffle the sounds of the surgical delivery)

__Wear your favorite scented lotion or perfume

__If you husband is your support person, have him wear his cologne, aftershave, deodorant, or other smell you prefer

__any ultrasound pictures you may have, favorite scriptures, inspirational quotes or affirmations, that you can read in the waiting room

__letters or cards written from other family and friends that you may have, to be read in waiting room

__pictures drawn by older siblings posted in room (and left with baby)

__incorporation of spiritual beliefs

The Welcoming

During this stage of pregnancy, you may likely be discouraged from seeing your baby. Your baby may not be delivered completely intact physically. If you ask your doctor during the time of the birth, you may be allowed to have your baby's physical form returned to you after their analysis/autopsy of the baby is complete. If you are permitted to have your baby returned to you, a representative of the hospital will likely call you within two weeks of the birth for you to come and receive your baby. He or she will likely be placed in a small container. Please know that your baby's physical form is not going to be intact, and this may be extremely upsetting for you to see. Please consider not opening the container.

Your doctor may also offer suggestions for physical pain relief, including medicinal options. You might also inquire of prescription of estrogen and progesterone treatments, as this has been theorized to reduce the incidence of intrauterine adhesions, therefore possibly preventing future additional fertility challenges as a result of the birth method needed for this pregnancy.

After the Birth

- Have the photo you brought placed with your baby.
- Have the blanket you brought placed with the baby (just leave these items in the room if you like).
- Name your baby
- *See the "Professionals/Volunteers" link at stillbirthday.com for additional services to consider.
- Perhaps consider having a friend spend the night with you.
- You will still have lochia (the remaining blood from inside the uterus, for about a week or less).
- Watch for signs of postpartum depression (PPD) or secondary vaginitus.
- Watch for warning signs including fever, pain, filling a maxi pad sooner than an hour (bleeding after a medically assisted birth should be minimal), clotting, or a foul odor. Please contact your provider immediately if you experience any of

these signs.Consult with your OB about TTC. Most will recommend waiting at least 6 weeks, just as in a full term delivery. We have information here regarding TTC (trying to conceive) and getting pregnant again.

- Be easy on yourself, your body, and on your recovery.
- Talk to your trusted spiritual advisor, your husband, and trusted mentors and friends about all of your feelings.
- *Visit stillbirthday.com for "Farewell Celebrations" and for "Long Term Support" resources.

Have at Home After Birth

___people ready to help!

___maxi pads (for lochia, you may have postpartum bleeding for about a week)

STILL BIRTH

This plan is specific to a 31+ week delivery, in which you may be required to stay overnight.
You may not be required to stay overnight. Ask your doctor for more information.

Things to Know:
- Because the first plan covers 2 different birth methods, specifics to each particular birth method will be noted.
- Cesarean has its own birth plan because it is so in-depth. You might consider printing both plans, in case your birth turns into an emergency Cesarean.
- This plan is appropriate for pregnancies about 31 weeks to 40 weeks or more.
- These plans do not include specific options you may wish to include if your baby may survive past birth, including possible resuscitation, ventilator use, medications and additional testing. You should consider including these things if there is a chance of your baby surviving for any additional time past delivery.
- If your baby is expected to receive care in the NICU, here is a listing of NICU specific resources and information.
- Some providers discourage parents from touching preemie babies receiving NICU care. This article can give more information on why that is, and what you may be able to do. The NICU experience *alone* can promote parents grief. Please

see our article on Identifying Grief to find information and support regarding grief but also the correlation between the NICU experience and grief/depression/PTSD.

- Within the first 24 hours after your baby has died, there may be an opportunity for you to decide on organ or tissue donation. Please discuss this *in advance* with your spouse and with your medical professional. Purposeful Gift is an organization founded by an SBD trained doula. You can also learn more by Googling "donor network (your state)" , finding your local OPO, or contacting your local organ donation center. Cord blood information can help you determine the likelihood of your donating your baby's cord blood. Here is information specifically for organ donation from an anencephalic baby. Any of these things will depend on a number of factors unique to your situation.

- Get more birth education and learn what to expect during labor, here.

- Please visit our link on general postpartum health (your emotional and physical health after delivery).

Helpful Tips:

- Check out our listing of local professionals and volunteers willing to support you through the process
- Learn about the special way to give a stillborn baby a bath.
- consider hand or feet molds of your baby
- consider inkless prints: fingerprints/handprints/footprints of your baby
- Your body is likely to produce breastmilk after the birth of your baby. Please learn about post loss lactation . This link discusses breastmilk donation in particular.

- If your state doesn't offer a birth certificate for stillbirth, consider printing off our unofficial birth certificate (found at the Farewell Celebrations link).
- Consider special farewell words or music.
- Also include a personalized farewell celebration.
- Ask for your ultrasound photos, or visit a local Crisis Pregnancy Center that performs ultrasounds, and ask if you can have one last photo of your baby.
- Prior to birth, if your baby still has a heartbeat, consider using your cell phone or other recordable device, and record the doppler's sounds of your baby's heartbeat. You can then add this to a Build-A-Bear as a momento. Alternatively, you can purchase a beautiful Angel Heartbeat Bear, which has everything included.
- Prior to birth, consider having a belly cast done as a momento.
- Prior to birth, consult with your doctor and with the funeral home that you select, to see if special considerations can be made, such as, you leaving the hospital with your baby, to take to the funeral home.
- More momento and special ideas are listed in the birth plan.

Have an idea of what your baby may look like. You can visit stillbirthday for photos of babies shared by mothers.

What to Pack

__ camera, stillbirthday.com lists professional photographers at the "professionals/volunteers" page.

__photo of you and your husband to keep with baby

__Clinging Cross or something special to hold

__*additional special items: two teddy bears or blankets (one to leave with your baby, and one to take home), mold for baby's hands or feet

__Music and player

__Favorite candle (in glass jar, for warmer)

__Personal fan

__Several wash cloths, for hot or cold compresses (optional-hospitals have plenty)

__Thermos of hot water

__Massage tools: rice packs, rolling pin, paint roller, oil

__Unscented and scented lotion

__Birth ball

__Pillows (1 or 2) and colored cases

__Change of clothes for labor partner

__Snacks for labor partner

__Gum or mints for labor partner!

__Husband's cologne, aftershave, deodorant, or other smell preferred by the mother (he'll wear it)

__Snacks for you: light snacking during birth, orange juice postpartum

__Suckers or other hard candy

__Lip balm

__Cell phone or calling card

__Loose change for phone or snacks

__Phone list for support people to join you for hospital visitation

__Ultrasound pictures, favorite scriptures

__*baby's outfit (for visitation through to final farewell/burial)

__Toiletries: contact case, shampoo, toothbrush, deodorant, etc.

__Night gown or robe (might get soiled)

__Going home outfit for mom (2nd trimester clothes)

Have at Home

__people ready to help!

__maxi pads (for lochia)

__nursing pads (and cabbage, sage tea, and decongestant for expedited weaning, or a hospital grade pump and storage bags/bottles for milk donation) There is more in-depth information regarding post-loss lactation, and ways to help dry quickly or to pump for donation, at stillbirthday, available on the same page that you printed this birth plan.

About the Birth

NOTE: While it can be safe to deliver a very early miscarried baby at home, with precautions such as those listed in the at-home miscarriage birth plan, delivering a stillborn baby at home can come with some complications. If you are adjusting this plan to deliver your stillborn baby at home, please first consult your local police department to make sure that you are in compliance with your state laws regarding at-home stillbirth. Please make sure that you have a professional midwife to support you, particularly one with stillbirth experience. Please know that there can be medical complications in a stillbirth delivery, just as in a "happy" birth. Infection, postpartum hemorrhage, and other medical concerns should be prepared for. You should not deliver your stillborn baby at home alone. The remaining of this plan will pertain to hospital stillbirth delivery.

Natural Options/Information

- IV, with option of Heparin Lock instead
- Blood pressure cuff
- Possible electronic fetal monitoring
- No food or drink
- Possible limited natural induction/augmentation and positions, because of risk of placenta pulling from uterus and causing internal bleeding
- Hands and knees on ball or on bed can be very helpful
- Left Side Lying can be very helpful

Ways of creating a soothing environment for birthing include (but definitely not limited to):

__dimmed lights

__soft music

__massage (scalp, feet, legs, back, even brushing teeth)

__inspirational messages and scriptures written on index cards or spoken aloud

__letters written from extended family and friends who can't attend the birth (read by husband)

__pictures drawn by older siblings posted in room (and left with baby)

__praying

__water therapy (bath until waters rupture, shower, misting spray)

__hot and cold therapy

__intimacy and bonding with husband

Artificial Induction Options/Information

- Possible cervical ripening agents (Cytotec-tablet or Cervidil-similar to a tampon applicator)
- Pitocin (possibly no water breaking)
- Likelihood of Epidural or Narcotic (Stadol, Nubain are examples)

Pitocin Information

+ Can start labor
+ Can speed up a slowed labor
+ Can increase intensity of contractions
+ Can stop a postpartum hemorrhage
+ Can be regulated and monitored closely
+ Can be turned off if necessary
- Difficult to produce natural progression of contractions
- Pain from Pitocin is often more difficult to deal with
- Requires IV and constant monitoring
- Mom *small* chance of hyptertensive episodes
- Mom *small* chance of titanic contractions
- Mom *small* chance of uterine spasm
- Mom *very small* chance of coma

Epidural Information

+ Catheter into epidural space in spinal column (1st space)
+ No need to repeatedly puncture: catheter can re administer or continue dosage
+ Given during Active labor (3-7cm)
+ Does not alter mom's consciousness
+ Can relax mom
+ Can help lower blood pressure of a PIH patient with high enough blood platelets

- **Goal of 80% relief, not 100%**
- Completely immobilizes
- Not administered promptly: same anesthesiologist for entire hospital
- Chance of longer second stage/ More difficult to push
- Mom chance of hypotension (drop in blood pressure)
- Mom chance of itching in face, neck and throat
- Mom chance of nausea, vomiting
- Spinal headache healed by patching hole with mom's blood
- Postpartum headache/backache
- Uncontrollable shivering
- Uneven, incomplete or failed pain relief
- Loss of perineal sensation: inability to push: increase cesarean chance
- Mom need catheter
- Mom chance of fever

Narcotic information

+ Given IV in Active labor (3-7cm)
+ Increases pain tolerance (doesn't eliminate pain, but takes "edge off")
+ Can be given ASAP
- Barbiturate derivative: anticonvulsive and hypnotic properties ("I feel drunk or something.")
- Wears off/ ACCLIMATION, need for increased dosage
- Can either increase or decrease labor (unpredictable),
- Can cause mom vomiting
- Can still feel highest peak of intensity, just not building up or let down

Simply ask your medical professional for the most up-to-date information on all options and how to receive comfort in conjunction to their recommendations for your safest experience.

Crowning/Delivery Options:

__I would like the use of a mirror to see the baby's head crowning

__I would like still photography

__I would like to be reminded and encouraged to touch baby's head while crowning

__forceps, vacuum or episiotomy may assist in final delivery of baby

__Umbilical cord may be cut by doctor *Can be cut "long" so that dad may "trim" it later.

These are extremely condensed versions of very basic information about medical options. It is so very important that you create a dialogue with your provider about what your options are, and what if any side effects you may experience, and how to receive support both for the birth and to ease any side effects of any support option.

After the Birth

__*Have the photo you brought placed with your baby.

__*Ask if baby can be swaddled in the blankets you brought.

__*Ask how long your baby can remain with you.

__*Ask if you can give your baby a bath.

__*Ask if your labor room or your postpartum room can be in a quiet location on the floor, where you have less of a chance of hearing other babies, or if you can be transferred to a different floor in the hospital. Transferring to a different floor means that you will not have maternity-specific care, however.

__*If your baby has hair, ask for scissors to cut a lock off.

__*Utilize all of the special plans you have, including saving mementos, holding your baby, capturing baby's smell with a blanket you will take home with you, dressing your baby, naming your baby, taking photographs, and including a pastor and friends and family.

See the "Professionals/Volunteers" link at stillbirthday.com for additional services to consider.

__Have someone planning on spending the night with you. Perhaps consider having a friend spend the night with you, so that your husband can go home, prepare the house, and rest.

__You will still have lochia (the remaining blood from inside the uterus, which will be shed for the next 4-6 weeks).

__*You may have breastmilk come in immediately after the birth. You can choose to pump and donate your milk, or go through the process of drying. Drying your milk supply can be done more quickly by drinking sage tea, taking a decongestant, and/or applying frozen or chilled cabbage leaves in your bra (until the soften and warm, and then change out). Expedited weaning takes about a week to complete. Some studies indicate that there may be a link between compounded postpartum depression and early weaning. More information regarding post loss lactation is available at stillbirthday, from the same page you printed this birth plan.

__*Mentally prepare for going home. The first few days at home can be very difficult.

__Watch for signs of postpartum depression (PPD) or secondary vaginitus.

__Be easy on yourself, your body, and on your recovery.

__Talk to your trusted spiritual advisor, your husband, and trusted mentors and friends about all of your feelings.

__*Visit stillbirthday.com for "Farewell Celebrations" and for "Long Term Support" resources.

*are specific to stillbirth

CESAREAN BIRTH
This plan is specific to Cesarean birth.

Things to Have:

__same sized clothes (at least one complete outfit)

__high sitting pants (not low cut), no zipper, no belt

__comfortable panties (high waist) may be more comfy than hospital issued panties

__open-bottomed shirts (no elastic around waist)
__scented spa eye sleep mask to cover your eyes in the bright operating room

__slip-on shoes

__Boppy or extra pillows

__ camera, since headphones are rarely permitted in OR, consider pre-recording a favorite song or songs onto your camera to play during prep/before the birth: doula also brings a camera, and stillbirthday.com lists professional photographers at the "professionals/volunteers" page.
__Clinging Cross to bring with you to the O.R.

__*baby's outfit (for visitation through to final farewell/burial)

__*additional special items: two teddy bears or blankets (one to leave with your baby, and one to take home), mold for baby's hands or feet

__there are things that you will not need to bring, that you will see listed at other websites and birth plans, including a carseat

<u>Have at home:</u>

__antacids

__Dannon Activia yogurt (for healthy digestion)

__journal (to remember when to take medications on time)
__high-fiber meals and soups
__people ready to help!
__items listed in this post: natural honey, Goldbond no-talc
__maxi pads (for lochia, and incision)

__nursing pads (and cabbage, sage tea, and decongestant for expedited weaning, or a hospital grade pump and storage bags/bottles for milk donation)

<u>The Process (Prep):</u>

You are not able to eat a certain amount of hours prior (to reduce risk of pneumonia).

The nurse may shave your bikini line (you can do this before labor begins).

You are given an antacid (again, to reduce pneumonia).

IV is set up.

Catheter is set up (it is removed the morning after). *If baby goes to NICU, you may not be able to get up to see her until the catheter is removed.

Blood Pressure, Heart Rate Monitor, and pressure boots (on legs) are in place.

Medicine is administered.

Brought to the Operating Room (possibly before this point). A paper sheet "screen" will block your view of the surgery, and your hands may be tied down to prevent you from spontaneously touching the open area. *Remember to bring your camera, a picture of you and your husband, and a few baby swaddling blankets to O.R.

The Medicine:

There are three ways the medicine adequate for comfortable and safe surgery can be administered.

Epidural: if you were already using this for labor, the nurse can add medicine appropriate for Cesarean to it.

Spinal: most common for Cesarean.

General: sometimes used for emergency Cesarean; no support will be allowed during birth.

You can ask your anesthesiologist about an analgesic that may allow you to be more alert after the baby is born (Duramorph).

Sensations from Medicine:

Instant, warm, tingly feeling in legs and chest (but some women report a "cold" sensation).

Instantly, the feeling of hunger is gone (a good thing!).

Warm feeling may change to cool if your blood pressure drops slightly.

May seem like you can't breathe. If you can talk, you're breathing. Hold your hand over your mouth so you can feel your own breath.

The Process (Birth):

Cut on skin (transverse "bikini cut" is most common)

Separate 6 pack muscle

Cut through peritoneum (a thin membrane)

Move bladder down slightly

Cut in uterus

Deliver baby! Any sensations of pulling or tugging are of the actual birth.

Umbilical cord cut by doctor *Can be cut "long" so that dad may "trim" it later.

Placenta released and removed.

*Baby swaddled, given to dad. Dad: hold baby close to mom's face, and ask the nurse to take pictures of baby, mom, and of you cutting (trimming) the cord.

The birth process can be completed in 5-15 minutes (the entire operation takes approx. 1 hour)

*Keep an extra camera with mom, with easy access to view newborn photos while remaining in Operating Room (may encourage quicker physical recovery).

*Have the photo you brought placed with your baby.

*Ask if baby can be swaddled in the blankets you brought.

*Ask if your baby can remain with you in the OR, or when you will be reunited in a Recovery Room.

*Ask if you can give your baby a bath in the recovery room.

*Ask if your recovery room can be in a quiet location on the floor, where you have less of a chance of hearing other babies, or if you can be transferred to a different floor in the hospital. Transferring to a different floor means that you will not have maternity-specific care, however.

*If your baby has hair, ask for scissors to cut a lock off.

Side Effects:

(common):

- Numbness (you will need to wait for the earliest signs of gaining sensations before moving to "recovery" room, which may be wiggling your toes or slightly lifting a leg—this can take 1-2 hrs)

- Soreness at medicine insertion site

- Ear ringing

- Shivering

- Anxiety

- Constipation

- Difficulty Urinating

- Headache

- Low Blood Pressure

- Nausea

- (other side effects):

- Skin Reaction

- Itching

- Pain at medicine insertion site

- Burning

- Inflammation

- Difficulty Breathing

The Process (Suturing):

("7 Layer Suture"):

- may heal faster

- Uterus stitched

- Bladder returned to place

- Peritoneum stitched (thin membrane around organs)

- Loosely stitch 6 pack

- Carefully stitch fascia (connective tissues of muscle fibers)

- Loosely stitch fat layer

- Skin sutures

("3 Layer Suture"):

- Uterus stitched

- Bladder returned to place

- Fascia carefully stitched

- Skin sutured

After the Birth:

Cesarean location (incision) will be covered in surgical tape.

You will remain in O.R. until you gain earliest sensations (wiggle toes or slightly lift leg) (1-2 hrs)

<u>Your Options (for Support People):</u>

You can have 1 person present with you during the birth (2 people is unlikely, but worth asking). That same person can stay with you in the Operating Room until you are moved to the "recovery"room on the maternity floor, where you will be reunited with your baby.

The person present for the birth can leave the OR after the birth, to go to your "recovery room" and set up your things and prepare the room for you. This person (your husband), and/or your other support person (doula) will most likely not be able to enter the O.R. after the delivery to support you, so you will not be accompanied by a support person again until you are moved to the "recovery" room.

In Recovery Room/Postpartum Room

It's called the same even for vaginal births. It's actually called "LDR" for Labor Delivery Recovery. After a few hours, you may be moved (again!) to a Postpartum room.

*Utilize all of the special plans you have, including saving mementos, holding your baby, capturing baby's smell with a blanket you will take home with you, dressing your baby, naming your baby, taking photographs, and including a pastor and friends and family. See the "Professionals/Volunteers" link at stillbirthday.com for additional services to consider.

Have someone planning on spending the night with you. Perhaps consider having a friend spend the night with you, so that your husband can go home, prepare the house, and rest.

You will still have lochia (the remaining blood from inside the uterus, which will be shed for the next 4-6 weeks).

For comfort, try putting a maxi pad between your underwear and the birth location (incision). Ask your doctor about adding Gold Bond (no talc) powder to the pad to keep the area dry, or Manuka honey on the incision to aid in it staying sealed .

Get propped up with extra pillows, use Boppy if it helps.

You may be prompted to walk sometime between a few hours to 12 hours after the birth.

Your catheter will be removed within the first 12 hours after the birth.

Gentle, careful movement is best. Walk for a few *minutes*, every few *hours* of the day for the first few *days*. This can actually help with the abdominal discomfort. Walk for a few minutes every hour of day after that (with doctor approval).

Get out of bed by first dangling your feet over, then move to a sitting position. Reverse this to get back into bed: sit on the bed first and slide into your pillow, holding the rail for support.

You may not be able to eat until you pass gas. Walking carefully may help this.

You might feel constipated, and may be given a stool softener.

Respiratory therapy may continue for the first couple of days postpartum. Holding your hands or a pillow over your incision area can help support it while you take deep breaths.

Narcotics are usually given for the first 12-24 hours after the delivery.

Take them correctly.

Pain medications are given after that. Take them correctly. Pain is easier to manage before it peaks—delaying medication can make it difficult to manage the pain.

Ibuprofin lowers inflammation=better healing and comfort.

*You will have breastmilk come in immediately after the birth. You can choose to pump and donate your milk, or go through the process of weaning. Weaning can be done more quickly by drinking sage tea, taking a decongestant, and/or applying frozen or chilled cabbage leaves in your bra (until the soften and warm, and then change out). Expedited weaning takes about a week to complete. Some studies indicate that there may be a link between compounded postpartum depression and early weaning.

Have husband or a journal to remind you when to take medications.

Rest. Healing happens when you sleep.

It can take 1-2 whole months for complete healing. Don't over-do it.

*Mentally prepare for going home. The first few days at home can be very difficult.

Watch for signs of postpartum depression (PPD) or secondary vaginitus.

Remember to stay connected to your spiritual support system as well.

Sensations (at birth location)

(worse in the first few days):

- Pulling

- Tugging

- Burning

- Aching

- Itching

- Red

- Puffy

- Uterus Cramping (even for vaginal births, as uterus is shrinking)

- Occasional Sharp Pain, in abdomen, chest, or shoulder area (may be from air entering abdomen during birth—a gas relief medicine may be recommended to get the air out)

Warning Signs

- Bleeding at site

- Oozing at site

- Site opening up

- Smelling bad at site

- Persistent pain

- Fever

- Difficulty breathing

Help Yourself Heal

(Massage)

- Find a massage therapist or physical therapist experienced with Cesarean recovery.

- Myofascial release techniques (gentle pressure applied above the affected area (feeling of tugging or bumpy)

- Cross Friction (Encourages proper formation of scar tissue)

(Other)

- Avoid stairs

- don't waste walking (keep things close)

- Lift nothing heavier than a few pounds

- Do NOT drive

- No sex for 6 weeks (same as vaginal birth)

- Your doctor may recommend not TTC for at least 6 months

- Drink water frequently

- Nap often

- Limit visitors

- Move gently, and as recommended (a *few* minutes every *few* hours at first)

- Listen to your body. After the first week, you may be able to stretch your body out a bit more, with pelvic tilts, leg lifts and other gentle stretches.

- Ask friends providing meals to prepare soups for easy digestion, or meals high in fiber to help with your intestinal movements.

- Be easy on yourself, your body, and on your recovery.

- Stay connected to your spiritual beliefs, your husband, and trusted mentors and friends about all of your feelings.

- *Visit stillbirthday.com for "Farewell Celebrations" and for "Long Term Support" resources.

FATAL DIAGNOSIS

This is an informational article on what to possibly expect to have occur from the time you discover a difficult diagnosis, through the birth, to the farewell celebration that you choose to honor your baby.

1. The very first consideration to make is in working through your feelings. You may experience any of these feelings, either immediately, or through the duration of your pregnancy, and these are not in any order. You need to know that other parents have come before you on this overwhelming journey, and they have felt these very same feelings:

- sadness

- anger

- disbelief

- disappointment/resentment

- jealousy of others

- shame

- shock

- acceptance/peace/even joy over your own pregnancy and child

113

Studies show that this "pre-grief", or "anticipatory grief", grief experienced prior to the actual death of your child, does not substitute the grief that will occur after your child dies. You will likely experience all of these feelings, and more powerfully, in the days, weeks and even years after the birth and death of your baby.

More information regarding grief and emotions can be found at our emotional/spiritual link.

2. You need to get support around you. Decide on who will walk this journey with you, and know that in most cases, your loved ones truly want to be a support to you, although they will likely feel ill equiped. They need their own resources and support, too, and it may take you to let them know that, if their questions become overwhelming and take away from the time you need to sort through your own feelings and experiences. Consider including any of the following people, or others:

- your parents and/or in-laws (Nothing Without You was started by a stillbirthday mother, who has resources for parents and for grandparents)

- closest friend(s) and family (guide them to the family/friends link)

- perinatal hospice support in your local area

- Alexandra's House or other prenatal and/or postnatal housing assistance and support

- professionals experienced with your baby's diagnosis in your area (including transferring prenatal care to a different doctor or hospital)

- other supportive professionals and volunteers in your area, like doulas and photographers (pregnancy/birth/farewell – listed at stillbirthday by state)

- bereavement support in your local area (visit the long term support services link)

- pastor

- professional counselor

- specific support groups or resources if this diagnosis indicates likelihood of future infertility, such as Hunter's Syndrome, Mitochondrial Disease, or Spinal Muscular Atrophy

- additional support services such as the cost of ultrasound provided by Sustaining Grace

- other moms who've come before you. You can read stories by clicking on "All Newborns/Diagnosis" in the right sidebar of this site.

- you can decide how you want to tell your loved ones. Starting a blog for your baby is a great way to work through your feelings, have a special online place that honors your baby, as well as allows others to see what's happening without seeming intrusive.

3. You are still pregnant, with a live child inside you. Your baby's experience in-utero is not totally conditioned on your perceptions or feelings toward your experience and this journey. However, it is important to come to find ways of celebrating this pregnancy and bonding with your baby now, while you can. Consider any of these things:

- prayer. It releases oxytocin, sending this oxygen-rich love hormone through your bloodstream to be received by your baby.

- connection with your husband, including sexual and non-sexual intimacy and togetherness. Getting a couples massage or retreating to a bed & breakfast weekend getaway in the country is a great idea.

- purchase a Build-A-Bear with personalized audio recording, to bring to an OB appointment with you. Record your baby's heartbeat, to be put in the bear.

- have a pregnancy belly casting done.

- have a Celebrating Pregnancy blessingway (Sacred Circle) with your closest friends.

- sing and talk to your baby, and touch your belly.

- journal, or write letters to your baby.

4. Prepare for the birth while you are pregnant:

- **view our birth planning information that includes information on lactation, NICU, and more.**

- consult with your OB over your hospital policies regarding infant death. Ask about:

- homebirth or other options

- the care that will be given to your baby. Are you planning on offering comfort care, or palliative, medical care? If your baby will receive intense medical support, investigate the possibility of delivering at your local intensive care children's hospital, to prevent a transfer of care after delivery.

- time you can have with your baby after delivery (any concerns or possible situations that would limit this)

- what to expect your baby to possibly look like (we accept donations from mothers of photos of their babies, so that mothers coming after you can help get an idea of what to possibly expect. Please submit photos to Heidi.Faith@stillbirthday.com and they will be added to the

"Gestational Age of Your Baby" tab, after all of the weeks of pregnancy photos.

- visit or call the maternity floor, and ask if there are nurses there with experience with babies with your baby's diagnosis

- rooming-in with your baby, kangaroo care/skin-to-skin bonding, breastfeeding

- ask if shots, ointments, and screening can be delayed or just not performed

- if your baby lives longer than expected and is able to leave the hospital with you, ask ahead of time what to expect in caring for your baby

- if your baby is not expected to live longer than your hospital stay after delivery, ask about making special arrangements to take your baby to the funeral home (if you can do it, or not)

5. Preparing for your baby's death now, while you are still pregnant, is very emotionally difficult, but it may allow you to create specialized plans for your situation.

- consult with different funeral homes, asking them what their experience is in infant death, and what special arrangements they might be able to offer in your specific situation.

- ask if they can arrange for you to bring your baby from the hospital to them.

- if they cannot do this, ask if, when they arrive to the hospital for your baby, if their representative can carry your baby out of the hospital in their arms, just like a live baby.

- see our Farewell Celebrations for additional suggestions.

Additional Support:

Books

Waiting with Gabriel

A Gift of Time

Empty Cradle, Broken Heart

More Books

Websites

Diagnosis & Surviving:

Down Syndrome Pregnancy

Medical Dwarfism

Fatal Diagnosis:

Cherishing the Journey

String of Pearls

Birth Plan **(from String of Pearls website)**

Growing through Affliction **(a letter from one mother to you)**

Special Needs Adoption

Madison's Foundation

Congenital Heart Support

Congenital Diaphragmatic Hernia Support

Congenital Diaphragmatic Hernia Support

Congenital Diaphragmatic Hernia Support

Trisomy Support (13 or 18 or related)

Trisomy Support (13 or 18)

Trisomy 18 support

Trisomy 13 support

Anencephaly support

Prader-Willi Syndrome Support

Spina Bifida Support

Cleft Lip/Palate Support (and related)

Prenatal Partners for Life

Be Not Afraid

Sufficient Grace

Waiting with Love

Beads of Courage

Project Sunshine

Purposeful Gift

Noah's Dad – raising a Down's Syndrome child from the dad's perspective

NICU support/micropreemie/preemie (scroll to bottom)

In addition, put these terms in your search engine to get even more support from your location.

Fatal Diagnosis Information

Prepare for the birth while you are pregnant:

· view our birth planning information that includes information on lactation, NICU, and more.

· consult with your OB over your hospital policies regarding infant death. Ask about:

· homebirth or other options

· the care that will be given to your baby. Are you planning on offering comfort care, or palliative, medical care? If your baby will receive intense medical support, investigate the possibility of delivering at your local intensive care children's hospital, to prevent a transfer of care after delivery.

· time you can have with your baby after delivery (any concerns or possible situations that would limit this)

· what to expect your baby to possibly look like

· visit or call the maternity floor, and ask if there are nurses there with experience with babies with your baby's diagnosis

· rooming-in with your baby, kangaroo care/skin-to-skin bonding, breastfeeding

· ask if shots, ointments, and screening can be delayed or just not performed

· if your baby lives longer than expected and is able to leave the hospital with you, ask ahead of time what to expect in caring for your baby

· if your baby is not expected to live longer than your hospital stay after delivery, ask about making special arrangements to take your baby to the funeral home (if you can do it, or not)

This plan is specific to your baby being born, and then dying during your hospital stay or shortly after birth. There are additional notes and options given, for a situation in which your baby survives longer than expected and may be discharged from the hospital with you. Whichever outcome you are expecting, it may be best to at least have some information regarding the other possible outcome.

You will find important information related to fatal diagnosis here.

You may want to print our extra time birth plan as well.

What to Pack

___ camera, stillbirthday.com lists professional photographers at the "professionals/volunteers" page.

__photo of you and your husband to keep with baby
__Clinging Cross or something special to hold

__*additional special items: two teddy bears or blankets (one to leave with your baby, and one to take home), mold for baby's hands or feet

__Music and player

__Favorite candle (in glass jar, for warmer)

__Personal fan

__Several wash cloths, for hot or cold compresses (optional-hospitals have plenty)

__Thermos of hot water

__Massage tools: rice packs, rolling pin, paint roller, oil

__Unscented and scented lotion

__Birth ball

__Pillows (1 or 2) and colored cases

__Change of clothes for labor partner

__Snacks for labor partner

__Gum or mints for labor partner!

__Husband's cologne, aftershave, deodorant, or other smell preferred by the mother (he'll wear it)

__Snacks for you: light snacking during birth, orange juice

postpartum

__Suckers or other hard candy

__Lip balm

__Cell phone or calling card

__Loose change for phone or snacks

__Phone list for support people to join you for hospital visitation

__Ultrasound pictures, favorite scriptures

__*baby's outfits (for visitation through to final farewell/burial)

__*several different folding-style hats and gauze for baby with cephalic diagnosis

__*organ and breastmilk donation and other things you may have decided – and the ability to change your mind about any decision at any time

__Toiletries: contact case, shampoo, toothbrush, deodorant, etc.

__Night gown or robe (might get soiled)

__Going home outfit for mom (2nd trimester clothes)

__a carseat, in the event that your baby survives longer than expected and can return home with you

Have at Home

__people ready to help!
__maxi pads (for lochia)

__any equipment that you may need in the event that your baby will survive a short time and be able to come home with you

__nursing pads (and cabbage, sage tea, and decongestant for expedited weaning, or a hospital grade pump and storage bags/bottles for milk donation) There is more in-depth information regarding post-loss lactation, and ways to help dry quickly or to pump for donation, at stillbirthday, available on the same page that you printed this birth plan.

Birth

Natural Options/Information

- IV, with option of Heparin Lock instead

- Blood pressure cuff

- Possible continuous fetal monitoring

- No food or drink

- No standing, because of risk of placenta pulling from uterus and causing internal bleeding

- Hands and knees on ball or on bed

- Left Side Lying

Ways of creating a soothing environment for birthing include (but definitely not limited to):

__dimmed lights

__soft music

__massage (scalp, feet, legs, back, even brushing teeth)

__inspirational messages and scriptures written on index cards or spoken aloud

__letters written from extended family and friends who can't attend the birth (read by husband)

__pictures drawn by older siblings posted in room (and left with baby)

__praying

__water therapy (bath until waters rupture, shower, misting spray)

__hot and cold therapy

__intimacy and bonding with husband

Crowning/Delivery

__I would like the use of a mirror to see the baby crowning (know that your baby's diagnosis may increase the chances of a face-first presentation)

__I would like photography

__I would like to be reminded and encouraged to gently touch baby's head while crowning (you should discuss this with your OB prior to labor)

__forceps, vacuum or episiotomy may assist in final delivery of baby

__Umbilical cord may be cut by doctor *Can be cut "long" so that dad may "trim" it later.

After the Birth

__*Have the photo you brought placed with your baby.

__*Ask if baby can be swaddled in the blankets you brought.

__*Decide if you would like to delay or forfeit all standard medical support after your baby is born and focus on bonding and time together, or if you would like standard medical support for newborns, including Erythromycin in her eyes, Vitamin K injection, bulb suctioning of her nose and mouth to clear the airways, and APGARs.

__*Decide if you want your baby weighed and measured.

__*Decide if you would prefer life saving medical support, including positive pressure ventilation, intubation or chest compressions, or if the focus should be on comfort.

__*Decide if you want pain medication administered to your baby in the event he or she is in pain.

__*Ask how long your baby can remain with you.

__*Ask if you can give your baby a bath.

__*Ask if your labor room or your postpartum room can be in a quiet location on the floor, where you have less of a chance of hearing other babies, or if you can be transferred to a different floor in the hospital. Transferring to a different floor means that you will not have maternity-specific care, however.

__*If your baby has hair, ask for scissors to cut a lock off.

__*Utilize all of the special plans you have, including saving mementos, holding your baby, capturing baby's smell with a blanket you will take home with you, dressing your baby, naming your baby, taking photographs, and including a pastor and friends and family. See the "Professionals/Volunteers" link at stillbirthday.com for additional services to consider.

__Have someone planning on spending the night with you. Perhaps consider having a friend spend the night with you, so that your husband can go home, prepare the house, and rest.

__You will still have lochia (the remaining blood from inside the uterus, which will be shed for the next 4-6 weeks).

__*You will have breastmilk come in immediately after the birth. You can choose to pump and donate your milk, or go through the process of drying. Drying your milk supply can be done more quickly by drinking sage tea, taking a decongestant, and/or applying frozen or chilled cabbage leaves in your bra (until the soften and warm, and then change out). Expedited weaning takes about a week to complete. Some studies indicate that there may be a link between compounded postpartum depression and early weaning. Additional information regarding post loss lactation can be found at stillbirthday, from the same page as this birth plan.

__*Mentally prepare for going home. The first few days at home can be very difficult.

__Watch for signs of postpartum depression (PPD) or secondary vaginitus.

__Remember to pray and ask others for help and for prayer.

__Be easy on yourself, your body, and on your recovery.

__Talk to God, your husband, and trusted mentors and friends about all of your feelings.

__*Visit stillbirthday.com for "Farewell Celebrations" and for "Long Term Support" resources.

WHEN GIVEN EXTRA TIME

The following information is specifically for babies who survive a longer time after birth:

When Given Extra Time

Provide breastmilk: Begin by pumping your milk, just shortly after the birth. Pump on a regular schedule even if you cannot give it to your baby right away (the hospital will help you store it), or even if milk doesn't come in abundantly. For different reasons, you may have a difficult time initially getting your milk to come in. Providing breast milk for your child is the one thing you can do for your baby that no one else can. Your baby may feed with a nasogastric tube, and can receive your breastmilk that way. Your breastmilk may actually provide a sort of "sterilization" to this tubing, because of the sIgA and other proteins present. You might consider introducing a pacifier after each tubal feeding, to allow your baby to associate suckling with being fed. Latching on can be difficult for babies who haven't yet developed the ability to suckle and breathe at the same time. Once baby latches on, he may eat often, but you will need to pump after feedings to empty the breast. You can begin feeding approximately every two-three hours after a good breastfeeding relationship has been established. Ask for help: utilize lactation support and contact the professionals around you for support.

These are tips to help breastfeed your baby, borrowed with permission from a mother whose experience is similar to yours:

As soon as possible, hold your baby skin-to-skin, also called "kangaroo care".

Pump as soon as possible, and for 20 minute sessions, every 2 hours; do not reduce this to less than 8 pumping sessions in a 24 hour period.

When pumping to increase supply, pump for a few minutes after the last drop.

When pumping to increase supply, consider "cluster" or "power pumping". Cluster pumping is pumping every half hour to hour for several hours. Power pumping is doing as absolutely minimal work but staying in bed and resting and pumping for 2-3 days.

As soon as possible, let your baby nuzzle your breast.

Don't overstimulate with rocking while they are trying to nurse.

Use the crossover hold.

Weigh your baby before and after a feeding, without changing the diaper. The grams gained are almost exactly equal to CC's of breastmilk.

Invest in a scale and an SNS for home (and Tommee Tippee breastflow—not drop-ins) . Your NICU nurse may give you an SNS for free. You can use an SNS and a nipple shield at the same time if you need to. Put the tube on your nipple (a little past the nipple on top), and roll on the nipple shield like a condom, give the SNS a squeeze to fill the nipple of the SNS and then latch the baby on.

Have your baby's tongue checked for tongue-ties and pallet issues.

Ask about cup feeding.

Ask about going home with your baby still on the gavage (see the study from Cochrane for more information.)

2. Bond with his caregivers: Natalie, the mother of a 25 week baby,

said, "Although you can't do a lot with a 25 weeker, it's nice to know how your baby is used to being handled by the nurses and doctors. This way, when you DO take over care, you can maintain consistency for your baby and help him/her to feel safe. In addition, knowing what was going on – in detail – helped me feel like I was getting to know (my daughter's) personality even though I couldn't interact with her the way normal mothers can. Like how much she liked to try to extubate herself, and how much she hated those wipe-down baths."

3. Talk to your baby: If you feel silly talking to a baby, read a book. It doesn't have to be a children's book – any will do! If you can't go to the hospital as often as you want, record your voice talking and singing to your baby. The staff can play it when you aren't there.

4. Hold your baby: Hold your baby as much as possible, but know that the earlier a baby is born, the more likely they are to be unable to tolerate touch. Touch can be painful or upsetting to the baby, and they show this by dropping their heart rate and oxygen levels. It's very hard, but those are your baby's cues that, just for right now, he wants to be left alone. Just as you would respect a term baby's cues to be left alone to sleep, you need to respect your preemie's cues.

5. Decorate his room: Bring in pictures from home – your older children, your pets, the grandparents. Bring in special stuffed animals and colorful blankets to cover the incubator. Make this "new home" as homey as possible.

6. Leave your scent: You, your husband, and your older children can

sleep with some soft cloth items and leave them for your baby. Large burp cloths and receiving blankets work especially well. You can pump with a burp cloth under your breasts so that any milk that drips can catch on the cloth, and then you can leave the cloth for him. Later, after he's had it for awhile, you can hold it close to smell your baby as you pump; his scent can facilitate a milk "letdown."

7. Dress your baby: As soon as the staff gives you permission, bring in his clothes. Don't worry if they don't fit perfectly.

8. Take pictures: Put together a little photo album to share with your friends. Your baby is a gift and should be celebrated!

9. Celebrate your baby: Find joy in his birth, and other "firsts", like his first bath or the first time he comes off of the vent. Take pictures and enjoy his tiniest, newest milestones.

10. Pray: Let the miracle of your child's life stay the priority while managing the conflicting and painful feelings of the experience. Get support, and keep an eye for signs of postpartum depression. Connect with other parents and with your church family and allow others to pray with you and share in the ways God is moving in the life of your family.

HOME STILL BIRTH

Understand your local laws regarding home stillbirth. Different state laws also provide for different regulations regarding stillbirth at home, particularly if there is a chance for survival. If your state laws permit you to have a home stillbirth, also determine if you have legal permission for any unique plans you have, such as burying your baby at a private cemetary. Your local officials can help you navigate your legal decisions.

Determine if homebirth will prevent life-saving or death-delaying medical support available from a hospital. If you know or even *suspect* that you may deliver a baby with a serious diagnosis but who also has even a slim chance of survival, you may decide to deliver your baby at a hospital, or discuss a transfer after birth with your midwife.

Consider any medical concerns that may impact your own health, including possible hemorrhage, uterine rupture, and infection. Discuss these risks with your midwife and make a plan to manage these.

Keep all diagnostic medical records from your pregnancy, including any ultrasound images that determine the demise of your baby. You will want to have these available at the birth, as your state laws may require you to present them to your local law enforcement official shortly after the delivery.

Work ahead of time with the funeral home of your choice. Learn their policies. Do they require arriving at your home to transport your baby to their facility? Will they permit you to transport your baby to their facility? Is there a timeframe from the time of delivery in which this transportation needs to occur?

Contact your local law enforcement officials at a responsible time after the birth, if this is included in your local laws (it likely is). They will need to see the diagnostic medical documentation that you've kept through your pregnancy, and ensure that you are safe. Please be respectful and comply with their questions.

Your midwife will need to have the official paperwork to submit to your local Vital Statistics office, to submit a request for an official Certificate of Death (this step may or may not be particularly difficult in your state).

To find ways of making your home stillbirth special, please consider viewing the hospital stillbirth plans as they may provide some support for you in your situation. Our birth education also has useful information.

Please visit the Farewell Celebrations section for support after the birth.

Please also consider sharing your story **of home stillbirth, and** read the stories of home stillbirth **from other mothers.**

Hydrotherapy is gaining increasing recognition as a homeopathic ingredient in birth planning.

Water can be included in labor and birth in a number of ways:

showering, allowing the water to splash onto your breasts and down your belly, to help stimulate labor

showering with your spouse to help increase oxytocin, to help stimulate labor

foot soak to ease tension and swelling

Waterbirth can take place at home, at a birth center, or in many hospitals. Contrary to its name, waterbirth not only means giving birth to your baby while you are emerged in water, it is also lesser understood to simply mean spending time soaking while in labor, whether or not the actual birth takes place while still emerged in the water.

Related: at home early pregnancy birth **and** at home stillbirth

Additionally, having a warm bath immediately after the birth can be soothing.

So, can a mother giving birth to her beloved miscarried or stillborn baby still enjoy the benefits of a waterbirth?

The answer? It depends on a number of very individualized and important factors, but YES, waterbirth may indeed still be a valid option.

If you have read through our birth planning materials, have consulted with your care provider, and desire to plan a waterbirth of your miscarried or stillborn baby, here are a few things to consider:

Including Epsom Salt at the measured amount directed on the carton can be particularly advantageous, for the following reasons:

Magnesium Sulfate is an FDA category A (good to know for mothers experiencing a threatened miscarriage).

Magnesium Sulfate can help reduce the risk of postpartum hemorrhage, a very serious danger which can be heightened for mothers giving birth via natural miscarriage.

Because hemorrhage is such a very serious and potentially life threatening issue for mothers experiencing pregnancy & infant loss, it is wise for you to consider that most generally during *any* water birth, blood released into the water can give an alarming appearance. Additionally, when you first stand up from your bath, you should do so carefully. Mothers giving birth in any trimester should *never do so alone.* Water and blood that has pooled in your vagina can also give an alarming appearance when you emerge from the water. Please be sure to read our information about hemorrhage because it is such a critical aspect of your experience.

Magnesium Sulfate has been used intravenously to stall preterm labor, but its actual ability to stall labor is inconclusive. In miscarriage labor, it is already possible for labor to start and stop over a timeframe up to weeks. Knowing this is helpful in your decision making.

Magnesium Sulfate can help fight infection because of its vasodilatation.

Soaking for 10 minutes at a time, in warm, fresh clean water, is recommended, when using Epsom Salt or not. This also helps to prevent reabsorption of your toxins flushed during the soak.

When you have high levels of stress, your body can deplete its source of Magnesium Sulfate, resulting in higher amounts of adrenaline production. These higher amounts of adrenaline can add to the already emotionally overwhelming experience of pregnancy and infant loss, and can even pose additional health risks. Soaking in a warm bath with Magnesium Sulfate can counter these dangers.

The saline water of your soak may aid in preserving the very delicate physical form of your miscarried baby. Using a small fish net to remove fragments of your baby's placenta from your bath may be helpful. Please see our at home birth planning for more information.

You might also add essential oils to your bath.

HOW TO BATHE A STILLBORN BABY

This article works in conjunction to our article that describes what to expect from the appearance of your baby, and the condition of your baby's skin. Please see The Skin of Your Stillborn for additional information.

Even the smallest of babies can benefit from a bath of sorts – babies born before ossification begins (approximately 16 or 17 weeks gestation and younger), can be gently placed in a clear container of saline water, which can allow the parents to hold and bond with their baby without damaging the physical form, and, this water can help restore a visible "fullness" of the physical form. You can visit our early pregnancy at home birth plan for more information.

Related: How to Photograph a Baby Not Alive

Caregivers often are concerned about showing a stillborn baby to the parents, because of the compromised condition of the baby's body. A baby who has been dead in utero for even a short time can have macerated and discolored skin and a misshapen head. Cleansing the skin of the compromised baby often may be viewed as adding more injury because the skin will slip even farther if a wash-cloth is used. The following information gives practical suggestions on how to care for a macerated stillborn infant.

1. Place the baby into a bath basin of warm bath water which has had baby shampoo added (I like to add Serenity essential oil).

2. Squeeze a washcloth with this shampoo water over the baby's body; do not rub.

3. With gloved hands, place baby shampoo in hands and gently glide over the stillborn's body to remove all drainage. Shampoo the hair gently also.

4. Next take the baby out of the shampoo water and discard the bath water. Rinse the soapy water off the baby by placing in a basin of warm water or by holding the baby under a gentle stream of warm running water from the faucet.

5. Take the baby from the rinse water and place on absorbent towels or underpads. Dab with a soft cloth, such as a Chix, to dry the baby – do not rub.

6. Place Vaseline gauze over macerated areas and hold in place with dry gauze wrap.

7. Transparent dressings (i.e. Opsite or Tegaderm) can be used over macerated areas if the skin next to these areas is intact. This type of dressing can be used over a weeping autopsy incision as well.

8. Dry ear canals and nostrils with Q-tips, gently.

9. If nostrils continue to seep fluid, place a small amount of petroleum jelly into each nostril. This will give shape to the nose and prevent further seepage.

10. Choose clothing that opens completely from the front or back. The important thing is to have clothing that promotes the least amount of handling and rubbing of the stillborn's skin. The least amount of handling prevents further skin slippage.

11. Parents appreciate their baby dressed in blue clothing for a boy

and pink clothing for a girl. Sometimes only blue or pink blankets may be available; use the appropriate color.

12. Diaper the baby.

13. Use a baby brush or comb to comb the baby's hair. A bow can be placed in a baby girl's hair by placing a small amount of petroleum jelly on the back of the bow to hold the bow in place. Give the comb or brush to the parents for a memento.

14. Snip a lock of hair from the back of the baby's head for the parents' baby book. Be sure this is within the family's culture or belief before providing this memento.

15. If the baby's head is misshapen, find a cap or hat that when tied under the chin makes the baby's face appear more round. Fill in areas of the hat with gauze or cotton balls if more roundness is needed.

16. When taking the stillborn baby to the parents, line the baby blanket with absorbent underpads so any further weeping can be collected in the underpad without saturating through the baby blanket. Spraying the underpads and the blanket with a commercial baby powder freshener gives a pleasant baby scent memory and lasts longer than baby powder.

How to Take Photos of a Stillborn Baby

17. Take pictures of the baby clothed and unclothed in uncluttered backgrounds. Sinks, garbage cans, cleansing equipment do not provide backgrounds for memories. Remember whatever you see in the camera viewfinder will be in the picture.

How to Position a Stillborn Baby in the Morgue

18. Positioning the baby in the morgue is very important. If the baby is not in good alignment with the head straight, pooling of blood occurs on the side of the face in which the head is turned. Proper positioning allows for subsequent viewings by the parents with little

change in the baby's facial appearance and color. Use diaper rolls around the head and remainder of the body to promote good alignment.

Related: How to Photograph a Baby Not Alive

Our stillbirthday birth & bereavement doulas offer guidance in bathing and more.

[Used with permission, RTS Counselor Training Manual, 1993, p. 132]

Care providers can provide positive memories even when the stillborn's skin is compromised. Hopefully, these tips will provide some practical ideas. For more information, please call or write:

Bonnie K. Gensch, R.N. RTS Bereavement Coordinator Lutheran Hospital—La Crosse 1910 South Avenue La Crosse, WI 54601 Phone: 608-785-0530, ext. 3796

(This article was copied in its entirety from WiSSP)

A Pregnancy Loss is Still a Birthday

HOW TO PHOTOGRAPH

Here are suggestions when photographing a baby not alive.

Photos as you enter the birth space:
- The parents' car
- The outside of birth place
- Nurses station or other signs to where the family are (maternity level or emergency room)
- The outside of birth room/room number
- Clock at intervals
- Parents after your introduction
- Any of their items/baby items
- Siblings or colorings from siblings (you can take a photo of their phone if they have any saved to that)
- Drinks, snacks, or other things that can serve to mark points of the labor, such as guests
- Parents – laughing, hugging, crying
- Crowning (hold in separate file for the mom)
- Early bonding
- As you leave, the clock or something outside to show the time change

To photograph the baby, here are some helpful tips:

- Begin taking pictures during pregnancy, the birth and as possible after birth. The physical form of the baby will change fast.
- Close-ups of the baby's hands and feet, and of the entire baby.
- You might include the parents' wedding rings, for size and to represent the special union which created the baby.
- You can include "props" like blankets, a flower or something meaningful to the family, and photograph the baby in different positions. A blanket can also be a beautiful way to cover parts of the baby with advanced physical changes while capturing a photo of hands or feet, for example.

Also Photograph:

- Every person impacted by the baby and present during whichever Season(s) you are capturing: Pregnancy, Birth, The Welcoming, The Farewell or The Healing Journey.
- Mom and/or Dad bonding with baby (reading, singing, touching, etc.).

During the Welcoming:
- Bonding.
- Actions including weighing & measuring.
- Items that touch the baby.
- Bathing and dressing.

Transitioning into the Farewell:
- Any keepsake making.

- Any staff present or parents on their phone.

Helpful tips about your camera, the photos, etc:

- Take time to read through and consider our pre-birth resource materials, including bonding in pregnancy, and creating the birth plan unique to this baby and this experience. These things can help create and capture meaningful events, feelings and experiences.
- Soften or shut off your flash. Using the light already in the room – window, computer screen glow, heat lamp, through the in-room bathroom, can be helpful.
- If you create both color and black and white copies, this lets the parents decide which they like.
- If you use editing software, keep copies of both versions so the family can choose. Trying to magnify the humanity of the baby while being realistic to what the family is actually seeing is important.
- Prepare the family to receive the photos – let them know you have them, and if possible, divide them between photos that can shape positive images of their experience, and the images that are more real, raw, or that you feel with your understanding of your time with them they may feel to be more private. These might be more graphic in nature. Hold a second copy of all photos in a safe place, for an amount of time you decide (1 year, 5 years, etc.), in the event that the originals become damaged.

If photographing the physical form of baby isn't possible:

- Perhaps in your birth experience, flushing was inevitable. The irretrievable birth of your baby's physical form into a bathroom basin can be for many mothers an extremely personal, painful and even traumatizing part of an already very painful experience. Please know that you are not alone. There are ways of speaking into this especially painful part of your journey with dignity and intention.

Perhaps purposefully including water into your farewell can be especially redeeming, such as a love letter to your baby into a beautiful stream or ocean.

- Photographing aspects of the reality of baby in other ways can piece together into a very significant photo journal. The pregnancy test, the nursery, a baby outfit, a special place that you thought of or think of now when thinking of your baby, even if these things are purchased and photographed after the birth and death of your beloved baby, can bring validation and healing.
- We have more keepsake and farewell celebration ideas.
- We have more support for during the birth here.
- We have both short term and long term bereavement support resources for you here.

Additional Resources:
- ADEC_article
- Digital Photography
- Midwifery Today

POSTPARTUM HEMORRHAGE

If you are giving birth at home, it is important to be aware of the symptoms of a possible hemorrhage.

Hemorrhaging is a serious concern in at-home miscarriage, and may be enough reason for your care provider to discourage you from attempting to complete your miscarriage at home.

Generally, you will probably be cautioned that filling a regular-absorbancy maxi pad sooner than one hour, at any time, is cause of concern; immediately postpartum (that is, right after the baby is born), generally speaking you should not fill a regular-absorbancy maxi pad sooner than a half-hour in the first hour (so, you can go through 2 pads in the first hour postpartum), as it is common to experience some increased bleeding at the actual time of delivery.

An at-home aid in reducing blood loss may be found in a small amount of apple vinegar. This is something best discussed with your care provider while you are still laboring and before the birth.

If at any time you fill a maxi pad sooner than a half hour, experience dizziness, or a racing heart, you should consult a medical professional immediately.

If you are soaking through a maxi pad sooner than recommended by your medical provider, you need to seek medical attention (if you cannot reach your provider, please go to your nearest emergency room) immediately.

Medications that may be prescribed to help control the postpartum hemorrhage include:

Misoprostol

Methylergonovine

Misoprostol (a prostaglandin) causes your uterus to contract, so that your baby can be delivered. In addition, the prostaglandin works to block a hormone (progesterone) from completing its pregnancy function of supporting the uterine lining that the baby has been growing in. This will stop your body's efforts of sustaining the pregnancy. "Cytotec" is one prescription name used, and misoprostol is said to have about an 80-90% effectiveness rate in delivering miscarried babies and completely expelling all of the placenta pieces. It is considered more effective than methylergonovine, but is not FDA approved for this use. For this reason, mothers may wish to request "Methergine" if it is considered a safer option by their provider.

Methylergonovine, commonly prescribed as "Methergine" is also a uterotonic; it causes your uterus to contract, which can shorten the duration of the delivery process, thus stopping the homorrhaging.

Your doctor will discuss with you the side effects and warning signs to look out for when taking these medications, and the amount of time it should take to complete the entire process.

Please visit our Levels of Augmentation article on herbal and natural alternatives to medications to help augment/speed up the time of the delivery of your miscarried baby.

(Click here to be taken back to the article on natural miscarriage or to the article on artificial induction.)

Postpartum (all birth methods)

It is important to take care of yourself, both physically and emotionally, following a pregnancy loss. Regardless of the kind of pregnancy loss or the birth method you've used, it is important to replenish lost vitamins from blood loss and the birth. Here are a few helpful tips:

Continue taking your prenatal vitamin.

Ask your provider about floradix, hemoplex or chlorophyll, as these are said to have nourishing properties that can aid in replenishing lost iron and providing additional oxygenation to your blood.

Stay hydrated.

Salty broths can be satisfying and aid in lost iron.

Vitamin C can help your body better absorb iron.

Getting sunshine (even a one time trip to a tanning spa if it's winter) can help invigorate you.

See the rest of our postpartum health tips.

DONATING BREASTMILK

Breastmilk is a gift of life.

Getting Started

- know the options for donating, including legalities and fine print (outside link).

- understand that the desire to donate alone doesn't make it happen. Sometimes even if there is milk, it is not enough or the mother's body doesn't respond very well to pumping.

- discuss with your provider about the possibility of a discounted hospital pump rental.

- purchase or rent a pump.

- purchase comfortable nursing bras.

- purchase breastmilk storage bags.

- learn how to exclusively pump (including storage, hand expression, cleaning tools, and more).

- create a word file within a tag or business card template as explained below for easier labeling.

· keep receipts for your purchases as they may be needed in your donating arrangement.

· get support from your loved ones.

· If you want to pump and save or donate you milk, you will need support. It can be very hard to find the strength to keep going, but your support can help you go for as long as you would like to.

KEY TIPS: To keep an adequate supply, so you will be able to continue pumping for as long as you want to, pumping at least 8-12 times a day is necessary. Pumping every 2-3 hours will keep your supply up. Pump for up to 15 minutes on each side – do not pump endlessly even with small amounts of milk as this can fatigue the breast and actually dry the milk. You may hold near to you, baby lotion or another scent, or an item that belongs to baby, to help with "let-down". Household support by friends, and awareness for you to give validation to your spouse in other ways (such as listening, hand holding) can soften the sense of guilt which may accompany the spouse's desire for you to stop pumping.

• Find a bra that fits. Once you start to pump, get a fitting to see what size nursing bra will fit.

Most maternity stores will size women, but if you don't want to go into a store with pregnant women and newborns, you can look up how to size it yourself online or you can ask for help from your doula if you're is comfortable with it. Another great option is nursing tanks or tank tops. They will keep nursing pads in place, and make it easy to pump yet give support.

• Look into a hands-free pumping bra. Here is one brand. These are invaluable. When pumping exclusively, mothers are stuck to a pump for hours a day, and holding the pump in place gets exhausting, especially since pumping is pretty boring. A hands-free bra will let you pump, but also let you read or work while doing it. To go along with this, pumping makes you lean over into an unnatural position, and there are flanges

(Pumpin' Pal) that go in the pump to lean the pump over while letting the mother relax.

• A good pump really helps ease the workload. If you would like to do this for longer than a month or two, you will need a pump that has the motor to sustain exclusive pumping. All hospital grade pumps will do this, though they are expensive. The Medela pumps aren't a closed pumping system so they aren't to be used for more than one person, but they are a good option. Hygeia pumps are the best pumps out there, and their professional grade pump are almost as powerful as hospital grade pumps for much cheaper. Ameda also has some amazing pumps to use.

• Drink a lot of water. Just the same as if you were nursing, you will need to drink water throughout the day to maintain her supply.

• Eat enough calories to stay healthy. One good rule of thumb is to eat 100 extra calories per 10 ounces pumped per day.

Pumping & Donating

• When storing milk, place the milk in whichever storage bag you have, and lie flat in your freezer until frozen. This takes up much less room in the freezer, so you can store more milk and it is much easier to transport. With some milk sharing arrangements, knowing on what day the milk was expressed is needed.

It might be simpler to create a word file with a tag or business card template that you can print multiple times, to include the following on each tag:

Your name, day that your baby was born, at what week gestation he or she was born at, and a simple blank space or line for you to write on the date you expressed that batch of milk.

If donating, find someone to donate to once you have a supply or milk stored. There are many places to look for families to donate to. Eats on Feets and Human Milk 4 Human Babies are communities run through facebook, and you can just do a facebook search to find the chapter closest to you. These are both direct donation communities, so the donation is completely up to the families involved. Most should cover any expenses you had, such as storage bags or shipping.

• It may take a few days for the supply to rise, since the body wasn't prepared to make milk as early as it did. One way to increase supply is power pumping. This is more time consuming than pumping, but it works really well. When pumping, you pump for 5-10 minutes, then take a 5-10 minute break. Continue this for about an hour to an hour and a half, even if nothing else is coming out of the breast. The stimulation, even if nothing is coming out, will increase the supply. You can do this multiple times a day to increase it faster, but it is time consuming.

Mother's Milk is an herbal tea traditionally used to increase breastmilk production.

• Make sure that the flanges fit the breast. A lot of women don't have the average nipples and breasts required to fit the standard flanges (horns) on the breast pump. Lactation Innovation http://bit.ly/pZCCAS is a great resource to see if the flanges are the right size. If they are too big or small they can cause a lot of pain while pumping, clogged ducts, uneven emptying of the breast, and other issues. Correct flanges will help pumping be much less stressful.

You will need support people, particularly a birth & bereavement doula, to be there, to check on you. It isn't easy to keep pumping, and there will be hard days when you may need someone to remind you why you started doing this. The benefits of breastmilk are endless, but after loss, it isn't that easy to remember why you started.

If you donate your milk, the first time you drop off milk or milk is picked up can be hard. Your friends or a doula can ask if you will need them there, just for support. It is your baby's legacy and a wonderful thing for you to do, but it was also to be your own baby's nourishment.

If you ever have any questions, please do not hesitate to contact any of our birth & bereavement doulas, or our lactation professionals. Kayce Pearson pumped after her second trimester loss for two months, donated over 1000 ounces to three families, and encountered a lot of problems along the way, from clogged ducts to issues wanting to continue. Anytime you need help, you can send her a direct email. Kayce Pearson heartsandhandsservices@gmail.com

Your loved ones will also need to provide support to you. They can:

- bring or prepare meals for you.

- help with some of your basic household chores (laundry, for example).

- help run errands for you.

- not expect you to "host" or "entertain" them.

·   visit our "friends/family" section for more helpful ideas.

·   encourage you that you are making the right choice for your
    needs.

·   remember that you are a new mom, which comes with a lot of
    needs, as well as a grieving mom, which also comes with a lot of
    needs.

Additional Information

This section is borrowed from "Expressing Breast Milk"written and
revised by Edith Kernerman, IBCLC, and Jack Newman MD, FRCPC,
IBCLC, and edited only to be appropriate for stillbirthday.

Obviously, if you can pump or express a lot of milk, you are producing a
lot; however, if you cannot pump or express a lot, this does not mean
your milk production is low or inadequate. Do not pump to find out
how much you are producing. This is not a good way to judge milk
supply.

The most effective pumps are high-powered, double, electric, and
hospital-grade with adjustable pressure/suction and speed. There are
many pumps on the market that are just not very good.   Some hand
pumps are adequate for occasional pumping.

Hand expression can be very effective and certainly is the least
expensive. See below.

Improper use of a breast pump can lead to problems. Read all
instructions thoroughly. Make sure you get a demonstration and
instructions from the person who is renting or selling you the pump.

Pumping Method

Wash your hands

Place your nipple in the center of the flange (when your baby is breastfeeding, it is best that your baby be latched on "off-centre" or "asymmetrically" with your nipple pointed toward the roof of baby's mouth (see the information sheet *When Latching* and the video clips.

Put the pump on the lowest setting that extracts milk, not the highest setting you can tolerate.

Pump for a maximum of 15 minutes each side. If breasts run "dry" before 15 minutes is up, pump until dry then add 2 minutes. Compression can be used when pumping as well and increases the amount you can pump. See the information sheet *Breast Compression*.

Remember, pumping should not hurt.   If it hurts:

> Lower the suction setting

> Ensure the nipple is centered in the flange

> Pump for a shorter period of time

Cleaning the Pump

All pumping equipment should be sterilized before first usage, thereafter it only requires washing with hot, soapy, water or by dishwasher.

After each pumping: either place the pumping kit (not the tubes or motor) in the refrigerator until the next pumping, or if not pumping the same day, hot-water wash and hot-water rinse well, then air dry.

Remember to take apart all pieces of the pump for cleaning—including the smallest pieces, and to ensure that no milk has clumped in the flange shaft.

Hand Expression

Many mothers find that hand expression is an efficient way to pump when only occasional expression is required. In fact, when colostrum is present and the milk production is not abundant (as normal in the first few days), it is often easier to get milk with hand expression than with a pump and many mothers find this the easiest way to express mature milk as well.

Wash your hands

Place thumb and index finger on either side of the nipple, about 3 to 5 cm (1-2 inches) back from the nipple.

Press gently inward toward the rib cage

Roll fingers together in a slight downward motion

Repeat all around the nipple if desired

Encouraging the milk ejection reflex (MER) or "let down" reflex

The milk ejection reflex or "let down" reflex is the sudden rushing down of the milk. Milk will flow quickly even if you are not pumping at the time. Some mothers may feel thirsty, sweaty, sleepy, or dizzy during a milk ejection reflex. However, many mothers do not feel this milk ejection response ever in their whole lactating experience. You do not need to feel or be aware of the milk ejection reflex in order for there to be milk. Some women only become aware of it after the first few weeks while others feel it only at the beginning and no longer do after the first few weeks. This has absolutely no bearing on milk supply.

You can encourage the milk ejection reflex by thinking about having your baby in your arms or at your breast or having a picture of your baby to look at or keeping a piece of his clothing next to you.

You may feel the milk ejection reflex or notice your breasts leaking or you may not. You are likely to pump more milk faster if you pump both breasts at the same time. Breast compressions, while pumping, can be very effective at increasing the amount expressed, it may be a bit awkward at first, but it can be done (mothers have fixed the cups so that they sit inside the bra and then use compressions) or the partner can do it.

Sharing the Legacy of Milk

Understand the pain medication options your providers might offer you and how these might interfere with your lactation options.

Undergo a screening like at a Milk Bank.*

Having a doula or friend with you, especially for your first drop-off is important, as well as having something tangible you might hold during the exchange.

About Milk Donation – Screening*

All donors to a HMBANA Milk Bank undergo a screening process that begins with a short telephone interview. Donor mothers must be:

- in good health

- not regularly on most medications or herbal supplements (with the exception of prenatal vitamins, human insulin, thyroid replacement hormones, nasal sprays, asthma inhalers, topical treatments, eye drops, progestin-only or low dose estrogen birth control products; for other exceptions, please contact a milk bank for more information).

- willing to undergo blood testing (at the milk bank's expense)

- willing to donate at least 100 ounces of milk (some banks have a higher minimum)

You would not be a suitable donor if you:

- use illegal drugs

- smoke or use tobacco products

- have received a blood transfusion or blood products (except Rhogam) in the last 4 months

- have received an organ or tissue transplant in the last 12 months

- regularly have more than 2 ounces of alcohol per day

- have a positive blood test result for HIV, HTLV, hepatitis B or C, or syphilis

- or your sexual partner is at risk for HIV

- have been in the United Kingdom for more than 3 months (1980-96)

- have been in Europe for more than 5 years (1980-present)

Donated milk is heat processed (pasteurized) to remove potentially harmful bacteria and viruses.

Join the SBD Milk Sharing Map

If you are sharing your baby's legacy of milk, if you are in need of breastmilk, or if you are a lactation support resource, you can list your information on our Milk Sharing Map.

SOURCE OF DOCUMENT:http://www.stillbirthday.com/2011/10/20/post-loss-lactation-2/

A Pregnancy Loss is Still a Birthday

DRYING BREASTMILK

In between the two options of donating or drying breastmilk, you may have even just a few droplets of breastmilk that you might save onto a cloth nursing pad, or create into a jewelry item, or, you may still be nursing an older toddler and can cherish the shared gift.

 The options for support and for validating your experience are many.

This following information comes as it's foundation from Kayce Pearson, SBD

• Do not bind off the breasts. This can cause clogged ducts and can lead to infection and mastitis. This includes tight bras like sports bras or tight tank tops.

• One of the best natural remedies is cabbage leaves in the bra. Just take regular cabbage leaves, either the entire leaf or cut since it needs to fit over most of the breast, and fit it in the bra. Make sure that if the entire leaf doesn't cover, put some on both sides of the breast. This will evenly decrease the milk supply without causing clogged ducts or any other issues. If this is done around the clock, most see a huge decrease within a couple days. Change out the leaves twice a day for the best effect. [preparing the leaves by cutting off the biggest veiny sections, and then placing them in freezer bags in the freezer, and changing them out once they become warm and soggy, can provide relief from the physical pain of engorgement as well as helping to dry the milk quickly.]

Ice can be your best friend. When decreasing supply, engorgement can happen. Using ice doesn't stimulate supply, and it helps take the edge off any pain they can be experiencing. Earth Mama Angel Baby makes Booby Tubes, which are great for this. They can be frozen or heated, and curl around the breast so all the sore parts are covered.

Earth Mama Angel Baby also makes No More Milk tea. Peppermint and sage also can help lower breastmilk supply.

Try not to stimulate the breasts at all. Any stimulation, such as rubbing in the shower, can signal the breasts to make more milk. However, if the breast is really engorged, hand expressing until comfortable can really help, as long as it isn't done every few hours.

FAMILY & FRIENDS

It can be terribly uncomfortable, wanting to offer support to parents of a lost child, but not knowing the best way to do it. Sometimes very well meaning and loving expressions can actually be received as insulting and damaging. To prevent this, here is a helpful list of ideas for you to consider:

Helpful Things You Might *Know*:

You can be a much needed support prior to, during (yes, that's right, during), or after birth in any trimester.

Research proves that the level of grief a parent experiences is *not* conditional upon the age of the child. Meaning, younger children are "worth" just as much grief as older children.

Mothers who experience pregnancy & infant loss are at risk of developing postpartum major depression. The risk of this depression is highest within the first six months after birth. **The mothers who are at greatest risk of becoming depressed are those who fail to show any signs of grief during the first two weeks after the birth** (source).

Experiencing pregnancy & infant loss in a way that demonstrates the reality of your baby's life, and death, is actually important to your postpartum health.

Men and women experience grief differently.
Supportive efforts might be helpful for one parent more than the other. We have support for dads here, too.

Grief can be ongoing, can seem unpredictable, and can take time. Parents remember their children for the rest of their lives.

You and your bereaved loved one may benefit greatly from you learning about their type of loss and the other information we share here at stillbirthday, including support for getting pregnant again, support for surviving siblings, facing a struggle with fertility, and more.

The parents at highest risk of complications in their emotional healing are those that show no signs of grief in the first two weeks following the death of their child.

The actual loss is only the beginning of a journey of grief. The four most difficult times following a pregnancy loss are often: the return of the first menstrual cycle, the month in which the gender of the baby would have been discovered, the due date for the full term delivery, and the timeframe of the first anniversary of the loss (first stillbirthday). Holidays within the first year can also be painful, particularly Mother's Day/Father's Day (and/or Bereaved Mothers/Bereaved Fathers days), Thanksgiving and Christmas. Mothers too can face climactic milestones in subsequent pregnancy and birth. It is extremely positive to remember these times and reach out to your loved ones during at least one of these, offering to share an afternoon together or just to let them know that you care.

Grief can include a full range of feelings, at any time, including happiness and relief. Grief isn't bound by blue or grey but can be every color of the rainbow.

You may be grieving, too, and may benefit from utilizing long term support services

If the couple has other children, there is information and support for older siblings.

Honoring the privacy of the parents is important, but so is being able to communicate your own grief. For that reason, we have a section here where you can share your story (and read other stories), and it will be published in the category of "friends & family". Your story can bless others in a similar situation, without overstepping the privacy that the parents may have requested. We ask that you *do not* use their real names in your story.

Grandparents grieve too. AGAST is one organization for grandparent grief.

Stillbirthday has helpful resources for **grandparents, fathers, surviving and subsequent children**:Emotional/Spiritual Support.

Crisis Lines, Books, Websites (some by country) can be helpful for you to know for the parents.

Helpful Things You Might *Bring*:

Bring A Love Basket, for the earliest and darkest days.

These are suggested items, and may be brought by more than one loved one:

buy a special gown (particularly from Bg&Co) for the mother to give birth in

gather information for the mother on prior to birth, during birth, and after birth

understand about postpartum items and support she may need, including maxi pads for lochia, and items to support her decision regarding breastmilk (including donation)

buy a small or medium sized package of heavy maxi pads for the mom (birth in any trimester can mean a lot of bleeding)

bring a meal (or two) that is easy to prepare (more information on this below)

bring healthful, easy to munch snacks that can aid in healthy grieving

buy a teddy bear or other gift, *particularly prior to or during the birth,* so that the mother won't have to leave the place of her child's birth empty-handed — see our craft idea with teddy bears below

give the mother a gift card (not a huge amount, $20 would be great) to her favorite shop or a clothing store

buy the mom a comfortably-fitting blouse that is *non*-maternity (especially if she was further along in pregnancy)

include a card that shares your sorrow and includes the baby's name, as well as lists any other tangible ways you are available to help, including babysitting surviving children, mowing, shoveling snow, folding a load of laundry or any other simple tasks.

Meal Tips:

Make enough for leftovers.

Consider the older children and their tastes. Including a McDonald's gift card can be helpful.

Write reheating instructions if necessary.

Bring a gallon of milk, a loaf of fresh bread and a fruit basket so that basic groceries aren't needed.

Do not send meals in a dish you need returned.

Call before you go.

Mailing a card with a restaurant gift card is a nice alternative as well.

These ideas and a beautiful story are shared at Cooker & a Looker

Other Helpful Things You Might *Do*:

Has your friend invited you to support her during the actual birth?
Learn some foundational tips on serving as a doula where birth & bereavement meet.

hire an SBD doula **or an** SBD chaplain

host a Celebrating Pregnancy blessingway /Stillbirthday Sacred Circle (*strongly recommended*, even if this is done after the birth of the baby)

consider our book list for loved ones in how to support through grief

consider our many keepsakes and jewelry items

buy a special gift acknowledging her loss (the comfort company has many ideas)

participate in any farewell celebration the family might be participating in

clean, tidy the home, do a load of laundry, bring in their mail, mow their lawn

attend any foll0w-up doctor's visits with the mom

talk about the baby by name

send a card to the family at the first birthday or another holiday. Lost for Words is one card line specific to pregnancy and infant loss, or a Birth Verse card

sign up for another grieving mother to send her hand written letters through the Joy Comes in the Morning project

buy a helpful book for the parents (see our list of books)

consider the mom's interpretation of your gestures

visit the Farewell Celebrations page, as there are gift ideas there as well

Honor the Dad & Other Children:

Our Momentos section has special keepsakes for Stillbirthday Fathers and Children.

Sharing our Fathers & Children resources could be very helpful.

Supporting the couple so that he is emotionally available to explore the birth and death of his child from his own perspective, rather than serving entirely in a protective role for his wife, is helpful.

Craft Idea:

Find out from the mother how much her baby weighs.

Measure out that weight in rice. If you don't have an ounce scale at home, bring your rice to the grocery store. Check in with a cashier or another employee first to be sure there isn't any confusion about theft or anything like that.

Measure out the weight in rice, using a small plastic baggie to hold the rice.

Purchase a teddy bear. A Build-A-Bear would work very well.

Carefully cut the back seam of the bear, remove a small amount of the stuffing, and place the baggie of rice into the bear. Sew up the seam.

Now the mom has a bear that weighs as much as her baby.

Incorporating a small pouch and zippered back as an alternative, to hold small keepsakes like the baby's hospital bracelet or a love letter to the baby, is also a loving idea.

Helpful Things You Might *Say*:

I want to know – in word or action, this could be the most important sentiment to convey. This individual mother, father or surviving sibling knows the most of their own experience, and coming alongside them in a way that is slow, that is curious, that is trusting, allows them to explore what the situation means to them, and allows them to express what the situation means to them. The most important thing you might say is nothing at all, but opening up a safe place to listen. You will not at all know how to come alongside this mother and this family if you do not take the time to know who this mother and family are – how do they interpret their experiences, what are their spiritual beliefs, what are their needs.

In our doula training, we teach this fundamental "series" of support: slow down, validate, provide options and supplement resources. To support well, you don't have to support alone. Be prepared to wrap the mother in support options and know of a few resources that match her needs.

I'm sorry

Your feelings are OK. (This might be followed with:) *If your feelings get scary or dangerous, a counselor or pastor can help you navigate them. I can help you find one.*

I don't know if she asks why it happened. Don't guess or assume.

I miss (name of baby) *too* or *I wanted to know* (name of baby) *too.* This should not be said in a way that suggests grief comparison or makes the parent feel guilty for "feeling too much", but should be said in a loving way of sharing the grief together.

If you have experienced a pregnancy & infant loss yourself, prior to fairly recent years:

In honor both of your own experience, and/or the recent loss that was experienced by your loved one, you may wish to join our mentorship program.

Your perception of care for pregnancy & infant loss may likely be very different than the care that is given today. You may recall any of the following in your own experience: not seeing your baby, not holding your baby, not naming your baby, not knowing where your baby was buried, not knowing if your baby was given his or her own grave. You may not have ever talked about your experience, although the pain and reality of the death of your baby is real. Please consider sharing your story with us. Your story will also be categorized in the "prior to 1990's" section if applicable.

MISS Foundation offers grief support for grandparents ("AGAST").

You may become jealous or confused at the care and attention that is given to mothers and families who experience loss today. There are positive, healthy ways to work through these feelings without projecting any negative feelings onto the couple as they endure their grief now. Please visit the long term support resources for ideas.

You can contact your local Vital Statistics office for information on your stillbirth experience so that you may have some deeper healing and closure to your own experience.

If you are pregnant, while a loved one is experiencing bereavement:

Consider sharing the news with your friend privately, and before you share the news with others. This allows her to process the information privately, and gives her control.

Acknowledge the very real grief that your loved one is enduring, and recognize that she may have many mixed feelings about your pregnancy. She may likely be genuinely happy for you, but this joy will likely be mixed with jealousy and hurt, and at different times in your pregnancy these feelings may be magnified. Validate to your loved one what you expect from her feelings, and let her know that she can discuss these things, either with you or with other support such as a counselor or pastor. Refer her to the long term support resources section for more information.

When planning your baby shower, discuss her invitation with her privately, preferably before the other invitations go out. Let your loved one know that she is invited and her presence will be meaningful to you, but that you acknowledge that it may be upsetting for her, and that you'd like to give her room to make her own choice regarding attending. She may like to give a gift separately instead of attending.

If you are a long distance from the family:

In addition to many of the above suggestions, Caring from a Distance has ideas you may be able to incorporate into your support.

If you are a provider:

Please visit our Provider Care section

If you have a social media page, you might use this logo

to demonstrate your support of families enduring pregnancy and infant loss.

You can retrieve it from the stillbirthday Facebook page.

Things That Would *Not* Be Helpful To Do Or Say

Things that would *not* be helpful to do:

remove, pack up, or destroy items from the baby room without both parents' permission

petition the mother in any way to celebrate anybody else's pregnancy or baby, until the mother initiates interest herself, or at least several weeks have passed

Things that would *not* be helpful to say:

One in Two Won't offers a little video, so that you can *hear* the things not to say.

Giving any explanation whatsoever (medical *or* speculation) is generally not a good idea.

Pointing out that the mother has more time to have children. Right now, she is grieving *this* child (and, conception may have taken longer than you know).

Pointing out that the mother has more children – either older siblings or multiples of the baby who didn't survive (unless her grief is becoming destructive, and more professional assistance is suggested to help).

Promoting the idea that a twinless twin is a singleton, for example, or that two surviving babies from a set of triplets are instead twins (seeming or attempting to ignore the reality of all of the multiples in the pregnancy).

Suggesting in any way that this is a positive or a good outcome.

Pressuring the mother or the father to grieve differently than they are. Please see our resources on different grieving styles.

Initiating or engaging in controversial discussions with either parent on topics such as elective abortion or some kinds of fetal research. This can serve to invalidate the grief the parent is experiencing – even regardless of their general or prior position on such topics. It may be wise to pick a different topic, or pick a different person to discuss it with.

Attempting to participate in decisions such as telling the couple they should start trying to conceive immediately, or offering discouragement at the news of a subsequent pregnancy.

Suggesting in any way that this outcome is the fault of the mother (or father), unless you are gently and compassionately offering support resources for an *obviously* risky situation that you *know* for certain occured during the pregnancy (ie drug abuse, domestic violence). Remember, offering general speculation is *not* a good idea.

Anything with *just*, said or implied, is hurtful. "You can just have more children, you should just get over it…"

Telling the parents where you believe their baby's soul or spirit to be can be received offensively regardless of their faith. Allow the parent the right to explore answers of life after death without belittling them or minimizing the reality of the death of their baby. In addition, attention to where the baby is, is only part of the care that a mother needs. It is extremely important to remember that *she is here* – she is *without her child* – and she is *hurting*.

179

A Pregnancy Loss is Still a Birthday

FAREWELL CELEBRATIONS

There are ways to honor your little one, regardless of just how little he or she is.

These ideas are specific to recognizing the life and death of your baby – at any time, including funeral planning and keepsake items to purchase from different organizations. There are also many personalized birth plan options to help you celebrate the life of your baby during the labor and delivery.

Celebrating

A very young, unrecognizable baby:

A baby not buried:

A baby from a long time ago:

Celebrating Pregnancy Blessingway – Stillbirthday Sacred Circles

SBD Chaplains have *many* special, unique alternative cremation and burial options. These can be very difficult decisions but it can be very important to know that you have options you may not otherwise know about. SBD Chaplains use tools and resources including small cast iron pots, fruit dehydrators and many more ideas that are available simply for you to consider.

placenta burial

unofficial burial (including baby clothing and casket information).

farewell words and music (can be included in the unofficial burial)

Using a *very* small piece of paper or colored tissue paper, you can draw a picture or write a note and flush that during the time of your bleeding. Or, you can release flower petals or a love letter to your baby into a stream. Many stillbirthday mothers value incorporating water into their farewell when flushing was inevitable.

Some funeral homes offer a memorial wall or garden for names of babies who are not buried there.

Confirm with your local crisis pregnancy center that they can and should offer ultrasounds for every mother *enduring an impending miscarriage*, as this may be the only photo she will have of her baby, and consider donating to their organization if they do offer such a valuable service to bereaved families.

Donate to your SBD doula or to our SBD doula sponsorship program to equip more doulas to serve families.

Donate to an organization or business that offers discounted or free pregnancy & infant loss resources (such as Mason's Cause or AngelNames.org).

Raise funds for your local perinatal or pediatric hospice/palliative care.

Volunteer to help minister to and encourage other mothers: here are important tips to consider when resolving to get involved.

Place a birth and/or death announcement in your local newspaper so that you can keep that for your own keepsake.

Create a birth or a death announcement (or both) in a postcard or other format. We offer an online version at stillbirthday.

Birth & Bereavement Activism, Art & Expression.

Blog about your story or in other ways reach out and share your experience.

Share your experience with us here at this site (we'd be honored and blessed).

Spread the word offers a "Blog Button" and other ways to help others including our Debris Day.

Order a stillbirthday cake.

Special remembrance jewelry (See our list! There's a lot!)

Special momentos (See our list! There's a lot!)

Release a balloon, perhaps with a small letter or prayer attached.

Please see our birth plans for a full section of birth planning, birth, and immediate postpartum support, including, for example, items from Earth Mama Angel Baby.

Purchasing an unofficial Certificate of Birth as a momento. Portraits by Dana offers one as well. (Stillbirthday has a free Certificate of Birth basic template).

Incorporating water into your farewell, particularly when flushing is inevitable:

Seashore of Remembrance

Sacred Water Offering

Celebrating

An identifiable baby:

An older baby:

Any of the above ideas for a smaller baby.

See your state listing of professionals/volunteers for photographers in your area.

Consider breastmilk donation (and get help from the hospital staff with nursing).

Investigate as soon as possible if your state offers an official certificate of stillbirth.

Visitation at hospital, home, or funeral.

Farewell words and music (can be included in the funeral).

Official, cemetary burial options (including hospital cremation, funeral home cremation, funeral, clothing, and casket information).

If you have baby items or the nursery already set up, do not pack anything away until both parents agree to this decision. If at that time you decide that you'd like to share your baby's items with others, Missing Solace has a Christmas present donation program. You can also participate in our Love Cupboard program.

Special momentos for older babies (see our list! There's a lot!)

Honoring Stillbirthday Fathers

Dads can honor the real life and the real death of their babies in special and unique ways, including any of the above ideas. For more suggestions, visit our:

- family and friends/ gift ideas for dads

- support resources for dads

Things that may *not* be very helpful

Believing or acting as though the burial location is a nursery or that the baby is somehow living there.

Volunteering for long-term projects in your baby's name, because if you cannot follow through you may be left with tremendous guilt.

Naming a pet or another child the same name as your lost child, unless both parents fully agree to this.

If you've experienced loss in the past

You may know someone who's lost a baby *many years ago*, and never thought there were options for their family to honor their little one. No time or distance can deter a mother from celebrating the life, and death, of her child. If you are that mother, you can still honor your child. You can choose from different items on this page, too, in particular, the ones for celebrating a very young baby.

Cultural Farewell Traditions & Customs

& Burial Items

Our SBD Chaplains can officiate the farewell celebration of your choosing, as well as guiding you in caring for your baby's physical form and preparing for natural burial. All of our SBD Chaplains are also trained SBD Doulas, which means that they can also support you prior to and during your birth, as well as support your postpartum needs. You can visit the "During Birth" resources for a listing of your local SBD Doulas and SBD Chaplains.

Burial Shrouds

Hindu

Muslim

Native American

Burial Jewelry

Baha'i

Matching Mother/Child Jewelry (one buried with baby, one kept and worn by mother)

Birth Verse

B'earth Angel

Cultural and religious information pertaining to bereavement (including cultural keepsakes) can be found in our Long Term Healing Perspectives section.

THE LONGTERM HEALING JOURNEY

The earliest moments of encountering the realization that your baby is not alive can be the most catastrophically overwhelming and quite literally the most traumatizing moments of your life.

This little booklet is only intended to place the most urgent and immediate options in front of you to consider as you embark on this difficult journey.

You are still a mother. You are still worthy of giving birth to your beloved baby, and your precious one will be born. If I can just encourage you with that, it would be that you are a beautiful mother, and that you matter.

Please, even in this impossible time, go slow.
Ask questions. Ask for support.

The experience of pregnancy and infant loss doesn't end when your baby is born. You will be for the rest of your life a mother. And for the rest of your life, you are worthy of healing.

When you are ready, make yourself a warm cup of cocoa or fresh lemonade, snuggle in your pajamas and pull up your computer. Type in www.stillbirthday.com.

The purple bar across the top of the screen guides you in chronological order, from support prior to birth – including explanations of medical terms, and what to expect from the birth method your medical provider deems safest for you.

The "during support" resources will lead you into hundreds of pages, similar to those in this book. Birth plan preparations including questions to ask your care team, information about alternatives and how to connect with a local doula, all are there.

Mothers who have embarked on this journey before you have allowed stillbirthday to hold their babies' photos, and their birth stories. From every week gestation to particular special and unique aspects of their stories, mothers, fathers, siblings and loved ones from all over the world have shared their stories at stillbirthday that you might know you are not alone.

There are events, news articles, research and interpretive resources for spiritual support and psychological understanding of bereavement, contributed poems, and more, all for you.

I am so very sorry for your loss and for what you may be enduring.

May you know simply that you are loved.

MY LONGTERM HEALING JOURNEY

Ways I have already grown:

_____

_____

_____

Areas I've forgiven others:

_____

_____

_____

Areas I've forgiven myself:

_____

_____

_____

New support I've discovered:

_____

_____

_____

Unexpected challenges I have met:

_____

_____

_____

Unexpected support I have encountered:

_____

_____

_____

Goals I have:

_____

_____

_____

MORE OF MY THOUGHTS

_____

_____

_____

_____

_____

_____

_____

_____

_____

_____

_____

_____

_____

_____

_____

_____

_____

_____

_____

_____

_____

_____

_____

_____

_____

_____

_____

_____

_____

FOR FURTHER EXPLORATION

There are numerous resources for support and growth through the journey of healing. Please take your time at stillbirthday to get to know the resources that are available to you – locally, nationally and globally.

Stillbirthday founder Heidi Faith has written a journal book that draws parallels to pregnancy and birth with being a bereaved mother, offering a guided journey through the gestation of grief, offering personal opportunities for exploration and learning how to both nurture your grief and set a healthy structure around it for your greatest growth.

The Invisible Pregnancy: Give Birth to Healing

ABOUT THIS BOOK

This is simply a compilation of the most urgent and immediate support and resources that families may need in facing the earliest moments of birth and bereavement. Please, visit stillbirthday for a much more comprehensive support – prior to, during and after birth in any trimester, and for support for the healing journey.

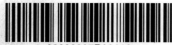

Made in the USA
San Bernardino, CA
23 December 2015